Celebrating 100 years of the Tavistock and Portman

The year 2020 marked the 100th anniversary of the first patient being seen at the world-renowned Tavistock Clinic. Over the following year, the Tavistock & Portman NHS Foundation Trust marked this centenary with a series of events celebrating its history and exploring issues of identity, relationships, and society. This book is a collection of essays from these celebrations, which describe the historical and contemporary work of various departments and services, and consider how to draw on this heritage to provide valuable responses to current and future challenges.

The twelve chapters describe the organisation's thinking, educational and clinical work with children, young people and their parents, adults, organisations, and wider society, documenting the influence of clinicians such as Balint, Bick, Bowlby, Garland, Glover, Malan and Pailthorpe. The authors outline the development of services for people who have experienced trauma, neurodiversity, complex and enduring mental health problems, and paraphilias or forensic behaviours. They address issues such as gender identity, the impact of couple relationship difficulties on parenting, systemic racism within the psychotherapeutic professions and the societal health inequalities revealed by COVID-19. The book concludes with a chapter exploring leadership and followership in organisations and how this can be applied to work in the NHS.

This book was originally published as two special issues of *Psychoanalytic Psychotherapy.*

Paul Cundy is a consultant adult psychotherapist and Psychodynamic Psychotherapy Lead at Northeast London NHS Foundation Trust, UK. He is an associate fellow of the British Psychological Society, Leicester, UK, and Editor-in-Chief of *Psychoanalytic Psychotherapy*.

Jessica Yakeley is a consultant psychiatrist in forensic psychotherapy, Director of the Portman Clinic, and Director of Medical Education at the Tavistock and Portman NHS Foundation Trust, London, UK. She is a fellow of the British Psychoanalytical Society, London, UK, and a former editor of *Psychoanalytic Psychotherapy*.

Celebrating 100 years of the Tavistock and Portman

Edited by
Paul Cundy and Jessica Yakeley

Routledge
Taylor & Francis Group
LONDON AND NEW YORK

First published 2023
by Routledge
4 Park Square, Milton Park, Abingdon, Oxon OX14 4RN

and by Routledge
605 Third Avenue, New York, NY 10158

Routledge is an imprint of the Taylor & Francis Group, an informa business

British Library Cataloguing in Publication Data
A catalogue record for this book is available from the British Library

ISBN13: 978-1-032-35145-2 (hbk)
ISBN13: 978-1-032-35148-3 (pbk)
ISBN13: 978-1-003-32552-9 (ebk)

DOI: 10.4324/9781003325529

Typeset in Minion Pro
by Newgen Publishing UK

Publisher's Note
The publisher accepts responsibility for any inconsistencies that may have arisen during the conversion of this book from journal articles to book chapters, namely the inclusion of journal terminology.

Contents

Citation Information

The following chapters were originally published in the journal *Psychoanalytic Psychotherapy*, volume 35, issue 4 (2021) and volume 36, issue 1 (2022). When citing this material, please use the original page numbering for each article, as follows:

Chapter 1
The Tavistock trauma service centenary lecture
Joanne Stubley
Psychoanalytic Psychotherapy, volume 35, issue 4 (2021), pp. 301–317

Chapter 2
Being safe and being brave: new thoughts on trauma, and adaptations to technique
Graham Music
Psychoanalytic Psychotherapy, volume 35, issue 4 (2021), pp. 318–334

Chapter 3
Trauma and abuse
Judith Trowell
Psychoanalytic Psychotherapy, volume 35, issue 4 (2021), pp. 335–352

Chapter 4
In the footsteps of Bick: continuing the legacy of infant observation
Dilys Daws and Alexandra de Rementeria
Psychoanalytic Psychotherapy, volume 35, issue 4 (2021), pp. 353–367

Chapter 5
Tavistock Centenary: the Tavistock Autism service over four decades
Sue Reid, Anne Alvarez, Nechama Polak and Myooran Canagaratnam
Psychoanalytic Psychotherapy, volume 35, issue 4 (2021), pp. 368–382

Chapter 6

Shapes of gender identity: three stories with impact
Domenico Di Ceglie
Psychoanalytic Psychotherapy, volume 35, issue 4 (2021), pp. 383–395

Chapter 7

Between partnering and parenting: psychoanalytic approaches to working with parental couples
Andrew Balfour
Psychoanalytic Psychotherapy, volume 35, issue 4 (2021), pp. 396–411

Chapter 8

Decolonising psychotherapy. Racism and the psychoanalytic profession
Helen Morgan
Psychoanalytic Psychotherapy, volume 35, issue 4 (2021), pp. 412–428

Chapter 9

Pandemic: challenges in care and recovery
Dinesh Sinha
Psychoanalytic Psychotherapy, volume 36, issue 1 (2022), pp. 4–12

Chapter 10

Under fire in the consulting room
Carine Minne
Psychoanalytic Psychotherapy, volume 36, issue 1 (2022), pp. 13–22

Chapter 11

The Fitzjohn's Unit
David Bell and Birgit Kleeberg
Psychoanalytic Psychotherapy, volume 36, issue 1 (2022), pp. 23–42

Chapter 12

'When I nod my head, hit it': leadership and followership in the orchestral environment
Lydia Hartland-Rowe
Psychoanalytic Psychotherapy, volume 36, issue 1 (2022), pp. 43–58

Notes on Contributors

Anne Alvarez, Consultant Child and Adolescent Psychotherapist, The Tavistock and Portman NHS Foundation Trust, London, UK.

Andrew Balfour, Psychoanalytic Psychotherapist, Tavistock Relationships, London, UK.

David Bell, British Psychoanalytic Society, London, UK; Consultant Psychiatrist in the Adult Department, The Tavistock and Portman NHS Foundation Trust, London, UK.

Myooran Canagaratnam, Consultant Psychiatrist in the Lifespan ASC and Learning Disabilities Service, The Tavistock and Portman NHS Foundation Trust, London, UK.

Paul Cundy, Consultant Adult Psychotherapist and Psychodynamic Psychotherapy Lead, Northeast London NHS Foundation Trust, UK.

Dilys Daws, Child, Young People and Family Department (retired), The Tavistock and Portman NHS Trust, London, UK.

Alexandra de Rementeria, Department of Education and Training, The Tavistock and Portman NHS Foundation Trust, London, UK.

Domenico Di Ceglie, Lifetime Honorary Consultant Child and Adolescent Psychiatrist, Founder and Former Director of Gender Identity Development Service, The Tavistock and Portman NHS Foundation Trust, London, UK.

Lydia Hartland-Rowe, Consultant Child and Adolescent Psychotherapist, The Tavistock and Portman NHS Foundation Trust, London, UK.

Birgit Kleeberg, British Psychoanalytic Society, London, UK, Consultant Adult Psychotherapist and Psychoanalyst, The Tavistock and Portman NHS Foundation Trust, London, UK.

Carine Minne, Portman Clinic, The Tavistock & Portman NHS Foundation Trust, London, UK.

Helen Morgan, British Jungian Analytic Association (BJAA) in the British Psychotherapy Foundation (BPF) Registered with the British Psychoanalytic Council (BPC), London, UK.

Graham Music, Portman Clinic, The Tavistock and Portman NHS Foundation Trust, London, UK.

Nechama Polak, Specialist Clinical Psychologist and Adult Psychotherapist, The Tavistock and Portman NHS Foundation Trust, London, UK.

Sue Reid, The Tavistock and Portman NHS Foundation Trust, London, UK.

Dinesh Sinha, The Tavistock and Portman NHS Foundation Trust, London, UK.

Joanne Stubley, Adult Department, Tavistock and Portman NHS Trust, The Tavistock Trauma Service, London, UK.

Judith Trowell, Consultant Child Psychiatrist and Psychoanalyst. Formerly of The Child and Family Department, Tavistock Clinic, London, UK and Health and Social Care, University of Worcester, Worcester, UK.

Introduction: Celebrating 100 years of the Tavistock and Portman

Paul Cundy

27 September 2020 marked the 100th anniversary of the first patient being seen at the Tavistock Clinic. Over the following year, the Tavistock & Portman NHS Foundation Trust marked this centenary with a series of events celebrating its history and exploring contemporary issues in relation to identity, relationships and society. This book is a collection of chapters based on presentations from the centennial celebrations. The authors, most of whom are past or present clinicians of the trust, describe the historical and contemporary work of various departments and services and consider how to draw on this heritage to provide valuable responses to contemporary and future challenges.

The Tavistock Clinic was established by Hugh Crichton-Miller, taking its name from its original location at 51 Tavistock Square. Crichton-Miller's aim was to provide civilians with the kind of treatments that he and other doctors had developed using Freud's theory of neurosis in the treatment of shell-shocked soldiers during World War 1. So, it seems fitting that the first three chapters in this book address the subject of trauma.

In 'The Tavistock trauma service centenary lecture' Jo Stubley describes the history and theoretical developments of clinical work with adult patients in the Tavistock Trauma Service. This service was founded in 1987 in response to the Herald of Free Enterprise Ferry Disaster. Using a psychoanalytic model of trauma developed by Caroline Garland, the unit initially worked with adults who had experienced a single episode trauma, offering a brief intervention of six consultations. However, over time, an increasing number of referrals have been received for people who have experienced chronic, repetitive and sustained traumas. Working with complex trauma has required changes to the original model, and advances in attachment and mentalisation theories and neuroscience have informed developments in the work of the unit. A range of therapeutic interventions, both individual and group, psychotherapeutic, physical and social is now provided.

The second chapter, by Graham Music, focuses on the developing field of trauma work, and the need to attend to the body. In 'Being safe and being brave: new thoughts on trauma, and adaptations to technique', Music describes his work with four young people to illustrate his journey as a trauma therapist, and the development of the techniques that he uses. Much of this requires a focus on the body, initially to develop feelings of safety and facilitate trust. Once this has been achieved the work can move towards emotional expression, again paying close attention to the body in order to regulate this experience. In doing so, Music is drawing on techniques from Intensive Short Term Dynamic Psychotherapy (ISTDP) developed by David Malan and Habib Davanloo. ISTDP offers a framework for understanding and working with body states, trauma and attachment, and can trace its origins to work that Malan began in 1956 as a member of Michael Balint's Brief Psychotherapy Research Group at the Tavistock.

An increasingly prevalent client group with complex trauma seen at the Trauma Service is people who have suffered historical (non-recent) sexual abuse. In the third chapter, 'Trauma and abuse', Judith Trowell reflects on how her work with this client group has been informed by an outcome study that was conducted more than 25 years ago to explore whether girls who had been sexually abused could benefit from psychoanalytic psychotherapy. The Tavistock was one of the organisations involved in this multi-site research project, which investigated the benefits of individual or group interventions offered to girls between the ages of 6 and 14 years and their parents or carers. The study revealed the importance of a settled family, and parents who could take the abuse seriously, to treatment outcome. Trowell links this to the availability of a protective and emotionally available object that can be accessed during therapy, and discusses this in the context of intensive long-term work with adults.

The Tavistock has provided services for children throughout its history. In 1920, the Tavistock Clinic was established with two departments: Adult and Children, and the first patient to be seen was a child. At the time having a separate children's department was quite revolutionary. Almost from the outset, education and training were part of the work of these two departments, as well as lectures to engage professionals and publicise the work of the clinic to the public. The next chapter describes an example of educational work developed at the Tavistock by Esther Bick, the psychoanalytic infant observation. 'In the footsteps of Bick: continuing the legacy of infant observation' by Dilys Daws and Alexandra de Rementeria brings the history of this technique to life. They describe three generations of teaching and learning infant observation, from Bick herself to the present day. The chapter goes on to describe clinical applications of the technique, such as consulting to a primary care baby clinic or a neurodisability clinic.

Neurodiversity is the subject of the following chapter, 'The Tavistock Autism Service over four decades' by Reid, Alvarez, Polak & Canagaratnam. Susan Reid and Anne Alvarez described their pioneering work adapting child psychoanalytic psychotherapy to meet the needs of children on the autism spectrum, at a time when the condition was little known or understood. They worked not only with these children but also emphasised the need to support their siblings and parents, their schools and wider networks. Nechama Polak goes on to describe how the service has worked more recently with adolescents and young adults, supporting them as they negotiate transitions. Myooran Canagaratnam concludes by reflecting on the recent establishment of an assessment service and how this has been shaped by the service's therapeutic roots.

Our next chapter, 'Shapes of gender identity' by Domenico Di Ceglie also describes work with young people, their families and their wider networks. Di Ceglie revisits three case studies to consider their influence on the creation of a model of care for children and adolescents with gender diversity. The Gender Identity Development Service (GIDS) was founded in 1989 at the Department of Child Psychiatry at St. Georges Hospital by Di Ceglie, to offer support to young people experiencing distress about their gender identity. In 1996, GIDS moved to the Tavistock and Portman NHS Trust, initially taking up residence at the Portman Clinic. Since 2009, the service has been nationally commissioned by NHS England and has grown in size and importance within the Trust.

The following chapter explores the link between couple relationship issues and parenting difficulties. In 'Between partnering and parenting: Psychoanalytic approaches to working with parental couples' Andrew Balfour describes psychotherapeutic work with parental couples at Tavistock Relationships. This organisation, which offers couple psychotherapy and practitioner training, has an approach that is rooted in psychoanalysis. It was founded in 1948 as the Family Discussion Bureau by social workers from the Family Welfare Association and psychoanalysts at the Tavistock Clinic, who shared an ambition to study the dynamics of family life. Tavistock Relationships' parent body, the Tavistock Institute of Medical Psychology, was incorporated in 1929, originally for the purpose of raising funds for new, larger premises for the clinic. Throughout its lifetime, Tavistock Relationships has been a 'sister' organisation to the clinic, sharing the distinctive 'Tavistock approach', with its focus on developmental challenges and developmental possibilities throughout the lifespan. Research evidence suggests that intense and unresolved conflict in the parental couple can be profoundly detrimental to their children's health, well-being and long-term development. Balfour describes how couples' psychotherapy can potentially be more effective than parenting programmes in resolving these difficulties for parents and their children.

In the same year that the Tavistock was celebrating its centenary, the world was shocked by the death of George Floyd. His murder sparked protests and marches in the UK, and several statues were pulled down. These statues were representations of historical figures linked to the slave trade, such as Edward Colston in Bristol. The protests have raised awareness of the UK's involvement in the slave trade, and the current problems of structural and institutional racism. In the next chapter 'Decolonising psychotherapy. Racism and the psychoanalytic profession' Helen Morgan investigates structural and institutional racism within the psychotherapy profession. She considers the defensive structures of disavowal within ourselves and our professional organisations, and the features of psychoanalytic training that produce a disabling complacency. These work against the radical changes that are required if the profession is to become one to which people of colour can feel they belong and that reflects twenty-first-century multicultural Britain. She concludes by offering some suggestions for ways of working against the racist assumptions behind some of our theories and our structures. The underlying conviction of the chapter is that this is a White problem, which White people need to address. It seems appropriate to turn our gaze away from the past 100 years and towards the future. How can we overcome racism within the profession – not only for the benefit of Black colleagues but because it also does harm to all of us.

Exploring the theme of inequalities, the next chapter is entitled "Pandemic: Challenges in Care and Recovery" by Dinesh Sinha. It has long been known that economic disadvantage is linked to higher rates of mortality and poorer access to healthcare (Black, 1982). More recent evidence has suggested that industrialised societies with the greatest income differentials (such as the UK and USA) have the poorest health and social development (Wilkinson & Pickett, 2009). The COVID-19 pandemic, which delayed the Tavistock centenary celebrations, has highlighted once again the inequalities in health within our society. Using the lens of everyday sadism, Sinha identifies corrosive and deliberate counter narratives to the themes of care and courage in this period. He describes how the pre-existing silos of separation between the privileged and dispossessed have prevented survival and wellbeing in the wider society. He cautions health and social care workers about the possible lapse into masochism and bravery as defences against exhaustion and the guilt of having survived when thousands of our colleagues have not. He highlights the need for awareness of our own feelings of guilt and aggression, so that they do not vitiate our capacity to care. Sinha suggests that the process of recovering from the pandemic is not just about the restoration of physical wellbeing but also the creation of healthier conditions in society that actively mitigate the scourge of everyday sadism.

The next chapter, "Under fire in the consulting room" by Carine Minne, describes her work with patients at the Portman Clinic. The clinic traces its history back to 1933, when the 'Psychopathic Clinic' was founded by Edward Glover at the West End Hospital for Nervous Diseases. It was established as the clinical arm of the Institute for the Study and Treatment of Delinquency (ISTD), earlier founded in 1931 as the Institute for the Scientific Treatment of Delinquency. The Institute had been inspired by the work of Dr. Grace Pailthorpe, a psychiatrist and psychoanalyst, who worked in Birmingham and Holloway Prisons. There, she became interested in the personality of women prisoners and in 1932 published '*Studies in the Psychology of Delinquency*'.

In her article Minne uses clinical vignettes with patients such as a woman who was convicted of infanticide. She illustrates situations when the therapist realised there was a sudden unexpected rise in the 'temperature' of a patient's mind. She likens this to the ignition of a fuse and discusses why this may have occurred. Minne relates this "ignition" to possibly premature interpretations, or a failure to notice how anxious the patient was in the presence of the terrifying object-therapist and also, patients' unexpected responses to external interferences during a session.

In 1948, on the creation of the National Health Service, the Psychopathic Clinic formally separated from the ISTD and became part of the NHS, renamed as the Portman Clinic. In 1970 it moved to its current premises on Fitzjohn's Avenue, next to the Tavistock Clinic. In 1994 the two clinics joined together to form an NHS Trust and then, in 2006, a Foundation Trust. For detailed descriptions of the history and development of the Portman Clinic, see Fishman & Ruszczynski (2007), Saville & Rumney (1992) and Shapira (2016). Today the Portman Clinic works with both children and adults suffering from problems arising from delinquent, violent or criminal behaviours, or paraphilias (disturbing and damaging sexual behaviours or experiences) either legal or illegal.

In another of her case examples Minne reports on her work with a man with a life threatening sexual perversion. Like many of the patients seen at the Portman Clinic, his behaviour can be understood as a compulsive need to act out an earlier unprocessed trauma. The focus of the treatments at the Portman Clinic tends to be on the clinician's affective experience of being with patients like this, who, by enacting their conflicts and impulses, create disturbed and disturbing states of mind in those around them, including their clinicians.

Minne describes how these situations unfolded during the sessions and reflects upon how they might have been diffused differently. She emphasises how best to maintain a psychoanalytic stance but also how to clinically judge when a session must be terminated in order to protect both patient and therapist from inadvertently ignited exploding 'bombs'. Minne stresses the importance of supervision and consultation with colleagues in managing this disturbing work.

The next chapter documents the history and work of the Fitzjohn's Unit, formed relatively recently in 2000. David Bell and Birgit Kleeberg provide a history of the development and work of this specialist service which delivers psychoanalytic psychotherapy for adults suffering from more complex and/ or serious disorders. The chapter describes the patients treated in the unit, many of whom have been unwell for decades. Using a variety of clinical vignettes the authors go on to illustrate the model of care and also more general considerations such as the nature of the psychoanalytic attitude and the relation of psychiatry to psychoanalysis. They conclude by considering the position of this work within the wider context of mental healthcare policy and provision in England and Wales. Huge shifts in the cultural and political landscape over the life of the Fitzjohn's Unit have resulted in the domination of the nomothetic perspective and the consequent industrialisation of healthcare provision. The authors describe how the Fitzjohn's Unit has been swimming against this current, trying to preserve and develop a different way of thinking about mental illness, human subjectivity, and culture in general.

We conclude this book with a chapter by Lydia Hartland-Rowe, entitled "When I nod my head, hit it': Leadership and followership in the orchestral environment". The chapter explores the parallels between leading and following in music settings, and leading and following in other organisational settings. Hartland-Rowe draws on literature from a range of sources exploring organisational life in the orchestra including organisational psychology, music education, social semiotics and sociology, and with reference to psychoanalytic and systems psychodynamics frameworks makes links between experiences of leadership and followership in the orchestra and work in the NHS. The modern NHS may be too large, too complex, and too pressured a system for an ideal model of leadership and followership to hold. But Hartland-Rowe describes the merit in identifying spaces where this way of approaching a shared task can be effective, and links this way of working to the psychoanalytic stance of 'not knowing'. She concludes that, like the orchestra when it is working collaboratively and with agreed structures for leadership and followership, perhaps we can transfer this capacity into our work in the wider organisation and system where we, like the orchestra, face the need to perform.

References

Black, D. (1982) *Inequalities in health: the Black report*. London: Pelican Books.

Fishman, C. and Ruszczynski, S. (2007) 'The Portman Clinic: an historical sketch'. In Morgan, D. and Ruszczynski, S. (eds) *Lectures on Violence, Perversion and Delinquency*. London: Karnac.

Saville, E. and Rumney, D. (1992) *Let Justice Be Done: The History of the ISTD – A Study of Crime and Delinquency from 1931 to 1992*. London: ISTD.

Shapira, M. (2016) 'Psychoanalytic criminology, childhood and the democratic self'. In Ffytche, M. and Pick, D. (eds) *Psychoanalysis in the Age of Totalitarianism*. London: Routledge.

Wilkinson, R. G. and Pickett, K. (2009) *The Spirit Level: Why More Equal Societies Almost Always Do Better*. London: Allen Lane.

The Tavistock trauma service centenary lecture

Joanne Stubley

In celebration of its centenary, The Tavistock and Portman NHS Trust hosted a series of lectures. This paper has evolved from a lecture on trauma work within the Trust shared with Graham Music. The history and theoretical developments of clinical work with adult patients in the Tavistock Trauma Service are outlined.

Introduction

The history of the Tavistock and Portman NHS Trust is inextricably linked with attempts to offer therapeutic interventions to traumatized individuals. Hugh Crichton-Miller, a neurologist, founded a charitable clinic in Tavistock Square in 1920 in response to his experiences of working with shell-shocked soldiers. By 1939 he was working alongside 90 honorary medical colleagues, clinicians who gave their time without pay in the service of offering psychotherapeutic interventions to the general public. It may be important to register that not so long before the development of the National Health Service, set up in the aftermath of the Second World War, the clinic required this kind of charitable support. This has links to our current-day situation where the Trauma Service relies on the support of many talented and dedicated honorary therapists, trained clinicians who offer their services for free to obtain expertise in trauma therapy. World War Two also saw Tavistock psychiatrist and army physician Wilfred Bion develop his understandings of group processes through his work with traumatised soldiers.

The history of the service and theoretical underpinnings

The Unit for the Study of Trauma and Its Aftermath was established by Caroline Garland and a group of Tavistock psychoanalytic colleagues in 1987 in response to the Herald of Free Enterprise Ferry Disaster. Originally the unit saw predominantly people who had been exposed to single episodes of adult trauma, often with diagnoses of Post-Traumatic Stress Disorder (PTSD). A brief intervention of a four session psychoanalytically informed consultation was the predominant therapeutic intervention at that time.

Garland's (1998) work with patients who had experienced a significant, single episode of trauma in their adult lives led to the development of a psychoanalytic model based on Kleinian theory. The notion of an internal world created through introjection of experiences with important others, along with phantasies and affects linked to these others allows for a recognition that all experiences are perceived unconsciously in terms of relationships. When a trauma occurs, regardless of the form it takes, at an unconscious level it is experienced as 'someone or something has done this to me'. And at the same time, 'my good internal relationships have failed to protect me and keep me safe'. Not only does the world become a dangerous place, potentially full of attacking, persecuting others, it is also a place where trust and the belief in significant others to keep one safe has been lost.

Powerful early anxieties linked to Klein's (1946) description of the early phases of infantile development which she called the Paranoid-Schizoid Position are re-evoked by trauma. These are life and death anxieties of annihilation, persecution, fragmentation and disintegration. It is a state of mind in which one's worst nightmares have been actualized. In order to bring order to this terrible, chaotic state, the ego attempts to find meaning in what is felt to be meaningless. It does so through an attempt to bind the traumatic experience to similar events that evoked these kinds of anxieties in the past. In the psychoanalytic model, we all have pockets of vulnerability, unprocessed traumas, losses and separations in which these kinds of anxieties were experienced and may never have been symbolized, thought about and mourned. Meaning at an unconscious level is given to the current trauma through the process of binding it to previous experiences – a way of providing a template – I have been here before and this is the relationship template that helps me to understand it. Illuminating and recognizing the unconscious meaning that is given to the adult trauma is part of the therapeutic work of the brief model Garland developed.

The model also focuses on the impact of trauma on the capacity to symbolize. Segal (1957) described symbolization as a function that requires a shift from Paranoid-Schizoid functioning to more Depressive position functioning. The capacity to use symbols is only possible if there is a recognition of the separateness of the other, acknowledgement of ambivalence and mourning of the loss of omnipotent control. Anxieties in the Depressive position are then more centred around guilt and remorse for the damage done to the other with the potential for reparation. Garland postulated that trauma attacks this symbolic capacity, and without words to think about what has happened, instead one is left with powerful anxieties and affects that push for action. One form this action may take is, through the use of projective identification, engagement in unconscious repetitions of the traumatic scenario in external relationships through the repetition compulsion. Freud (1920) described the way in which there is a pressure to re-enact the trauma when the capacity to 'remember' is impaired. Remembering in this context includes the ability to think about and reflect on the emotional experience of the trauma, including the capacity to bear the affects of grief and mourning that this will entail.

All trauma involves loss. This may be the more visible loss of home, loved one, or damage to one's body. There are also less obvious losses such as the loss of trust in the essential goodness and safety in the world or in the view of oneself. Bearing the annihilatory anxieties that are part of the response to trauma involves a recognition of one's own mortality. Since all trauma is experienced unconsciously as a relationship, there is a need to recognize the extent of human aggression and destructiveness, both in terms of what is perceived as having been done to you but also the reciprocal wish for revenge and the aggression this entails. Acknowledging this also involves loss of the previous view of oneself and the world.

Many of the individuals seen for the brief trauma intervention were stuck in a central paradox seen in trauma of endless re-living whilst at the same time being unable to remember and mourn what has been lost. Thus, mourning had often been impaired and the essential work of finding a way to move forward in life after a traumatic event had not occurred. The work of mourning also requires acknowledgment of the unconscious meaning given to the traumatic event – the previous experiences that evoked similar anxieties. What makes these events available for binding between past and present to occur is often that the earlier losses have not adequately been mourned. They remain unresolved and form pockets of vulnerability that later trauma may then blow open.

In the therapeutic encounter, the action of the repetition compulsion displays itself through the transference. The development of psychoanalysis using transference as a vital tool was enhanced by an understanding of the countertransference. Paula Heimann (1950) describes how the analyst's unconscious communicates with the unconscious of the patient and is noticed by attending to the analyst's feeling state. In turn, this has led to an elaboration of the concept to include what Betty Joseph (1985) describes as the total transference. In this, she describes the way in which much of what may occur in the therapeutic encounter may be understood as a transference communication that the analyst becomes aware of through close monitoring of their own state of mind and affective experience. The emphasis here is on the inevitability of much of the communication occurring at a non-verbal level.

The pressure on the analyst to take part in and be drawn into the transference, to act out with the patient, becomes the basis for enactments – moments within the therapeutic encounter where the patient and therapist become caught up together in acting out an aspect of the patient's unconscious drama, a drama that calls for action through the repetition compulsion. For traumatised patients, the pressure for action is particularly powerful for a number of reasons. The impairment in symbolic capacity, the failure to mourn losses, and the presence of powerful anxieties and defences from the paranoid-schizoid position all make action more likely and this is often in the form of the repetition compulsion (Freud, 1920). When Freud emphasizes the distinction between remembering and repeating through action, we understand this as capturing the complex process of what remembering entails – the capacity for narrative and affective experience as a prelude to the possibility of mourning. Thus, traumatised patients unconsciously construct a theatre within the therapeutic encounter in which the traumatic scenario may be endlessly repeated with the different roles of victim, perpetrator, witness and rescuer offered to others who may be drawn in. Therapists, almost inevitably, find themselves repeatedly and unconsciously pulled into such re-enactments of the traumatic scenario in its various forms. One only begins to have a sense of this through a close observation of the countertransference and a capacity to begin to reflect on the various ways in which one finds oneself responding to the patient.

Trying to bear what is being communicated, without action or attempts to be rid of it, is the beginnings of containment. Wilfred Bion (1963) described this notion in terms of mothers and babies. In the normal course of development, a baby is filled with the early, powerful anxieties I described earlier, and employs projective identification to communicate what is unbearable to mother. It is her role to try to take this in, to think about it and attempt to understand what might be going on in the baby's mind so that she might relieve him of his distress. Over time, this gives the baby the experience of someone who can mostly bear what they feel is unbearable and thus can lessen the need to rid oneself of distress.

The Tavistock trauma service

These psychoanalytic theories are particularly helpful in guiding an understanding of work with traumatised patients and were central to the model developed by Garland. They have also been seen as central to the model that we have subsequently developed within the service as our patient group has moved from Posttraumatic Stress Disorder (PTSD) to Complex PTSD. Whatever modality we are using and whatever stage of therapy we are working in, these theoretical concepts are the supporting structure that enable us to have a way of thinking about what is happening in the here and now in the room. What is at the centre of our work is the use we make of a psychoanalytic understanding of the impact of trauma, and the way in which the transference and our countertransference experiences help to inform us about our patient's state of mind.

Since the unit was established, there has been a gradual change in the kinds of referrals we have received. Many more traumatized asylum seekers and refugees, including victims of torture, have been referred. Their experiences are usually of a chronic, repetitive and sustained nature. We have also been referred veterans from the armed forces who have often had significant trauma prior to their wartime experiences. We are increasingly referred patients who have experienced significant childhood trauma, often with a recent adult trauma as the precipitant for referral. In the last few years, many of our referrals have been for historical child sexual abuse. Many of these different groups of patients would fulfil the criteria for Complex PTSD, whilst some may present with Dissociative Disorders, including Dissociative Identity Disorder. Other diagnoses may well be present – Depression, Anxiety States, Eating Disorders, Bipolar Disorder, Substance Misuse and Dependence, Personality Disorder, particularly Emotionally Unstable (Borderline) and so on.

It is also important to note that for some individuals seen in our service, the diagnostic labels they have been given within psychiatric services have potentially been re-traumatising in themselves. This is particularly true for the diagnosis of Emotionally Unstable Personality Disorder (EUPD), previously known as Borderline Personality Disorder. The message in these terms can easily be heard as 'there is something wrong with your personality, with you' and this is particularly problematic when childhood trauma can so readily cause a child to feel blamed, guilty or somehow bad. Although initial research (Cloitre et al., 2014) suggests there may be differences between the diagnoses of EUPD and C-PTSD, there is also a broader question to consider in relation to the impact of the Personality Disorder diagnosis on traumatised individuals. Coupled with this, the organisation of services around different diagnostic categories, such as eating disorders, personality disorders, substance abuse and so on can fail to engage with trauma as the central feature, contributing to fragmentation of care in individuals who may already feel fragmented.

As the impact of trauma, particularly early relational trauma, is becoming clearer, it is also challenging the traditional psychiatric classificatory systems. The use of a diagnosis based on symptomatology, even within a multi-axial framework, fails to capture the complexity of trauma-related disorders. A psychotherapeutic formulation that outlines the biopsychosocial elements to the presentation, I would argue, allows for the best evidence-based practice in relation to the trauma-related disorders. In gaining an understanding of the neurobiological, trauma and attachment theory research, current trauma-informed care requires a psychotherapeutic formulation that addresses the multiple ways in which trauma may have impacted upon that individual and how best to offer interventions in response to this.

This also links in with the Power Threat Meaning Framework developed by Johnstone and Boyle (2018) which highlights a trauma-informed exploration of an individual's distress and difficulties based on an exploration of what has happened to them, what meaning and narrative did they ascribe to this and what did they have to do to survive. It thus moves away from a medical framework and contextualizes an individual's responses within the complexities of their lives.

Judith Herman (1992) first used the term Complex Trauma to describe a constellation of symptoms that occurred following chronic, repetitive or prolonged trauma. She highlighted that the central feature of the experience was of captivity, being unable to escape from unbearable experiences of helplessness, terror and dread that overwhelmed existing defences. She drew on her clinical experience in working with adult survivors of child sexual abuse, Vietnam veterans and those individuals who had experienced domestic violence to suggest that for many the end result was characterized by a particular presentation of difficulties.

We have recognised the need to adapt and develop a model of working with these complex trauma patients that differs from the original model developed by Garland but remains, at its heart, informed by these psychoanalytic ideas. In working with and designing a service for individuals with C-PTSD we have also undertaken important and significant deviations from the original thinking. In essence, these differences centre on the position one takes theoretically in relation to the recognition of the external world – the trauma- versus the internal world – psychic reality and unconscious phantasies. Of course, there is always a delicate balance in attempting to hold both in mind but whilst a more traditional psychoanalytic approach would tend to favour a leaning towards psychic reality over the trauma, we would posit that a recognition, validation and attendance to the trauma and its impact is required in balance with the unconscious phantasies and this may necessitate a significant adaptation to the psychoanalytic way of working in order to engage with and work therapeutically with C-PTSD patients.

Over the years of developing the service, we have also had the considerable and growing literature from neurobiological, attachment and mentalisation theory. The introduction of the National Institute for Health and Care Excellence (NICE) led to treatment guidelines (National Institute for Clinical Excellence, 2019) developed from research evidence-based medicine and required service staff to train in modalities that were approved as first-line treatments for PTSD. I will describe this further later in this paper.

At the time of writing in 2021 the Tavistock Trauma Service now offers individual adapted psychoanalytic psychotherapy, trauma psycho-education groups, Eye Movement Desensitization and Reprocessing (EMDR), Narrative Exposure Therapy (NET), trauma art therapy groups, specialist Historical (non-recent) Child Sexual Abuse groups for women, young women and a planned group for men, Trauma-Mentalisation (MBT) groups, trauma yoga groups and a trauma gardening group. I will describe these further throughout the paper.

ICD 11 (The eleventh edition of the International Classificatory System of Diseases) includes a diagnosis of Complex PTSD (C-PTSD). Having a diagnostic category which brings together the experience of relational trauma with the potential impact on an individual's internal state and relationships allows for clear guidelines for care and a growing evidence base to draw on.

The International Society for Traumatic Stress Studies (ISTSS) have produced recommended guidelines for the treatment of C-PTSD based on best available evidence to date (Cloitre et al., 2012). Clearly, with a formal diagnosis still relatively new, the research evidence base is small. However, most experts recommend a phase-based approach to treatment which mirrors the original recommendations made by Herman many years ago.

These phases have been adapted by ISTSS to now include:

(1) Phase one: stabilisation (establishing safety, symptom management, improving emotion regulation and addressing current stressors)
(2) Phase two: trauma processing (focused processing of traumatic memories)
(3) Phase three: reintegration (re-establishing social and cultural connection and addressing personal quality of life).

Although perhaps less formally focused than the ISTSS guidelines, we would tend to also recognize something of a phase-based approach in our service, with the following headings:

(1) Therapeutic engagement
(2) Remembrance and mourning
(3) Therapeutic endings and reconnection

We would not see the phases developing in a clear linear fashion but rather as a guide to enable potential structuring of individualised treatment packages which recognize the necessity to adapt to where the patient is. This also accords with more recent research which questions the need to have a formal stabilization phase for all patients. (Cloitre et al., 2011).

The patient journey

Therapeutic interventions in the Tavistock Trauma Service thus hold in mind the phase-based approach whilst recognizing that what is essential in the work is the therapeutic relationship. The encounter begins with a four-session consultation, as designed by Garland; sessions of 75–90 minutes in length spaced at fortnightly intervals. This is not a consultation in the traditional sense but rather seen primarily as an opportunity to engage the patient in the therapy. Of course, within an NHS setting there are inevitably also a number of features that we need to ascertain, such as level of risk, whether it is possible to work within the boundaries of an outpatient service, the degree of relationship impairment – social isolation versus traumatic repetitions, the presence of dissociation and hyperarousal, and so on. Unlike a general psychotherapy assessment, the primary aim is not to elucidate the anxiety/defence structures with techniques designed to uncover these, but rather to focus on engaging the patient, establishing the groundwork for trust and to prepare the patient for the therapeutic work. We are also not using a capacity to work within the transference as a guide to 'suitability' since this is often not the case with our patients when they begin work with us. In time, this may become possible, but part of the initial engagement phase is to stabilise, support and strengthen the patient's resources and the therapeutic relationship to ascertain whether the second phase of trauma work will be possible.

Trust and engagement

Trust is a central issue in trauma. As Garland notes it is the loss of trust in our good internal objects to protect us that is as much a feature as the persecutory attack by bad objects. In early relational trauma, trust in attachment figures to protect and care is broken by the abuse. Luyten et al. (2019) links this to the notion of Epistemic Trust, the development through the caregiver relationship of a capacity to learn through social relationships, to recalibrate the world in the context of what is conveyed within the relationship. Many traumatised patients come to therapy with Epistemic Mistrust – a hypervigilance to threat and a difficulty in engaging with other minds to discover other perspectives and ways of viewing the world. This is linked to the development of disorganized attachment and failures of mentalisation, thereby perpetuating a state in which the expectation of the world as a threatening, potentially traumatising place is powerfully held. Daniel Taggart (unpublished communication, 2021) speaks of the need for the therapist to earn their 'trustworthiness' within such a relationship, emphasizing that the therapist needs to actively work on this rather than the onus being primarily on the patient to learn to trust.

Attachment research demonstrates a strong correlation between the disorganized pattern of attachment and childhood trauma (Main & Solomon, 1990). As Liotti (2011) describes it:

> *Being exposed to frequent interactions with a helplessly frightened, hostile and frightening, or confused caregiver, infants are caught in a relational trap, created by the dynamics of two inborn motivational systems, the attachment system and the defence (fight-flight) system. The attachment and the defence systems normally operate in harmony (i.e., flight from the source of fear to find refuge in the proximity to the attachment figure). They, however, clash in such a type of infant – caregiver interaction where the caregiver is at the same time the source and the solution of the infant's fear. (p129)*

The child is thus caught in a repetitive loop of approach – avoidance conflict, which may become a positive feedback loop, intensifying the distress. Neither approach nor avoidance works as a means of self-organization or as a way to alleviate fear. There is a collapse of the coping strategy and young children in these circumstances are not able to find a way to regulate affect. Lyons-Ruth (2001) describes how these disorganized babies and young children find an organizing strategy to cope with their disorganized attachment style by becoming either compulsive caretakers of their parents or aggressively bossy and hostile. It is a way, she postulates, of side-stepping the attachment system through the use of increasingly polarized and false-self relations with the caregiver. Taylor et al. (2000) calls this the 'tend and befriend' response –

a way of developing extreme sensitivity to the state of mind of the other and anticipating their needs and desires in order to protect oneself. As adults this may manifest in a hyper-alertness and sensitivity to others' states of mind and the ability to regulate themselves only by regulating others. The initial therapeutic encounter thus provides a potential space in which this kind of impact of relational trauma on current relational engagement can be observed.

With these thoughts in mind, the four-session consultation provides more space than a usual consultation (in the NHS usually 1–2 sessions) to begin to engage. Coupled with this, if patient and therapist feel they can work together, they would generally continue to do so after the consultation has ended. This may initially continue on a fortnightly basis, which often allows the patient time and space to manage the potentially threatening closeness and to titrate the amount of contact they can bear. It is then negotiated between therapist and patient when and if they move to once weekly.

Neurobiological studies have helped in our understanding of the difficulty in engagement in therapy for traumatised individuals. Early trauma has been strongly linked to heightened amygdala responsiveness to emotional faces especially threatening ones (Tottenham et al., 2011). Thus, the expectation is one of threat, and the threat is picked up through observation of the other's affective state. Coupled with this, there is often reduced anterior cingulate and orbitofrontal cortex volumes and connectivity which is associated with the dopamine reward system. In essence, if there is early relational trauma, it is an adaptive response to expect threat and not to anticipate reward. The difficulty comes when the environment changes to relative safety, for instance in therapy, but the system is set for an unsafe environment. Mackin et al. (2019) describe how the reduced reward system responsiveness coupled with reduced salience of positive social cues leads to reduced approach and increased aversion to others, heightening a sense of threat and seeing others as more likely to be untrustworthy.

This recognition of the importance of the enhanced threat system activation is used in the notion of the 'window of affect tolerance', first described by Siegel (1999) to describe the shifts between hyperarousal (fight/flight – Sympathetic Nervous System) and hypo arousal (freeze – Parasympathetic Dorsal Vagus). Siegel suggested there is an optimal zone between these two states where a person can be calm and focused, able to use their higher cortical, executive functions. This is the window of tolerance and in traumatised individuals this window will often be narrow. The awareness of the activation of the autonomic nervous system as part of the threat response is an important factor to be kept in mind in the engagement phase. The fight/flight response of the sympathetic nervous system may manifest itself through muscle tension and movement, an increase in respiratory rate with shallower breathing, trembling, sweating and so on. The freeze response is activation of the parasympathetic nervous system leading to hypo arousal – the body shuts down in the freeze response and this is generally associated with dissociation.

Dissociation

Dissociation as a defence in early relational trauma was powerfully described by Ferenczi in his classic paper 'Confusion of Tongues between the Adults and the Child – the Language of tenderness and passion' (1932/88). He describes how sexual abuse may lead to the dissociative response, emptying the mind so that identification with the aggressor can then occur. Ferenczi's use of this term is to describe how the unconscious identification works to allow the child to 'know' the mind of their attacker, to ascertain what is wanted, needed and desired as a way of protecting oneself. Dissociation has been neglected within the British Psychoanalytic Society, much like Ferenczi was early on after his split from Freud over this very topic. I would suggest that without an understanding of dissociation, working with traumatised patients can be problematic to say the least and this is reflected in the central position it occupies in many of the writings by the Relational Analytic group.

Trauma elicits dissociation which is a discontinuity of experience and memory. Allen (2001) describes it as having two components:

(1) Detachment from the overwhelming experience
(2) Compartmentalisation of the experience.

Dissociation is initially an adaptive response to terror and psychic pain, perhaps best described as the escape when there is no escape. When significant childhood trauma occurs, dissociation is likely to be triggered whenever the threat response system is activated.

In the early phase of engagement, one is also observing the patient's narrative. The Adult Attachment Interview studies demonstrate that those with unresolved trauma and loss will likely show this in their narrative, often with gaps, inconsistencies, avoidance or excessive preoccupation with the traumatic experiences. This links with the impaired symbolic capacity described by Garland. Indeed, neurobiological research now supports this finding, with evidence in early relational trauma of impaired functioning in Broca's area, the centre for language and the corpus callosum, which facilitates left–right brain connections, allowing for the affective experience (right brain) to connect with the narrative (left brain). Without words for experiences that have by their very nature provoked profound feelings of terror, dread and helplessness, the trauma remains unmentalised (Fonagy et al., 2002), unformulated (Stern, 1997) or perhaps most aptly described by Bollas (1987) they take the form of the 'unthought known'. As part of the dissociative process these experiences are often compartmentalised, hived off from other experiences and may only be evident in the incompleteness of the separation. This might lead to auditory hallucinations, anxiety reactions, recurrent nightmares, inexplicable somatic sensations and so on.

The trauma is thus held in the body – unsymbolised and dissociated from conscious awareness. Hence Bessel Van der Kolk's (2014) aptly named bestseller 'The Body Keeps the Score'. Recognising the importance of the body in trauma is an important part of understanding what adaptations to analytic work may be needed, especially in the early phases. Psycho-education groups offered alongside individual work allow for an understanding of the window of tolerance and the impact of trauma on this. Resourcing patients to recognize when they are feeling under threat and are entering hyperarousal is the first step in being able to counter this through techniques such as breathing exercises. Recognising the early signs of dissociation may then allow grounding skills to be employed. These resources, alongside the understanding of trauma that psychoeducation provides, empowers the patient to recognise their own responses, to listen to their bodies and to begin to be more present in the room. Unless a patient is within their window of tolerance, any intervention will be limited because at that point, the communication is essentially in the nonverbal realm.

Symbolic capacity and the body

The understanding of the impact on symbolic functioning in trauma work has also led us to offer a one-year trauma art therapy group, which we would see as a space to begin to bring what has been unnameable and perhaps unknowable, into the conscious mind through a medium other than words. This also links with our use of a trauma yoga group as an adjunct to the individual therapy, a compassionate space where reconnection with the body and a way to listen to one's body and what it has had to hold becomes possible.

These ideas also link in with an Attachment and Mentalisation approach to working with trauma. Early relational trauma may lead to epistemic mistrust, with associated impairments in attachment (particularly disorganized attachment) and failures in mentalisation. The development of epistemic trust within the mother–infant relationship is linked to nonverbal communications such as ostensive cueing and marked mirroring, which prepare the infant to be open to receiving social communication that is of relevance to him. This is an essential building block for mentalisation to develop within a secure attachment. Within the therapeutic relationship, the development of epistemic trust requires a sense of being recognised and understood, being seen for who they are and much of this is likely to be taking place within the nonverbal as well as verbal level of communication. Thus, traumatised patients from a mentalisation perspective need to begin therapy within a space that does not challenge or confront what they may not be fully aware of in order to build the relationship to enable mentalisation to begin. In recognition of this, we have recently begun offering trauma mentalisation-based therapy (MBT) groups within the service which run alongside individual therapy that is usually offered at fortnightly intervals.

The MBT work also links with a psychoanalytic understanding. Making an interpretation (particularly a transference interpretation) to a patient who is functioning in a traumatized state is unlikely to be taken in and reflected upon. It may be experienced instead as an intrusion or attack or intensify anxieties about not being listened to or understood. At this initial stage, the therapist's task may be more one of non-interpretative interventions as described by Holinger (1999). These might include clarification, mirroring, acknowledgement and validation. Joseph (1992) described how patients may come for understanding (being able to use the analytic space to reflect upon and consider their difficulties in the context of the transference) or they may come to be understood (to feel the analyst can connect with their difficulties and make sense of them). The first is much more depressive position functioning and the second more paranoid – schizoid. Many traumatized patients will be in the 'to be understood' category and even then, the wish for this may be small compared with the loss of trust and the belief in the goodness of the world they have experienced in response to the trauma. This emphasizes that the therapist's task at this point is to observe, reflect and attempt to engage with the patient. Joseph also spoke about the need to keep interpretations small, short and to the point when patients are struggling to think, to symbolize.

Stephen Porges' Polyvagal Theory (Porges, 2011) has helped us to understand the impact of trauma on the body and to link this specifically to the importance of relationships. It also serves to highlight further adaptations to psychoanalytic ways of working that may be required. As we have already seen, the threat response leads to automatic activation of the Autonomic Nervous system in either fight/flight (hyperarousal) or freeze (hypo arousal and dissociation). Porges highlighted that a component of the parasympathetic nervous system, which he called the Ventral Vagus Nerve has a different action. This is the most evolutionarily advanced component of the system and links the brainstem, heart, stomach, other internal organs and facial muscles. It is involved in complex processes of attachment, bonding, empathy and social communication. It is engaged when we socially connect with others through positive facial expressions, the tone and prosody of voice and so on. Thus, from the moment we greet a patient for our first encounter, we can elect to attempt to engage their Ventral Vagus Nerve, their social engagement system, through a warm, ordinary welcome. Of course, this may still cause activation of the threat system but is less likely to do so than the more traditional and reserved analytic stance.

External realities

An aspect of trauma therapy at any stage but perhaps particularly so at the initial stage of engagement is a consideration of external realities that may impinge on the work. ISTSS guidelines describe the initial phase as focusing on safety and stabilisation. If there are significant external issues, such as unstable housing, financial concerns, employment problems and so on, these need attending to. We have been fortunate to have trainee social workers join the service to help us address these often complex issues but it is also an important aspect of the therapy that the therapist recognizes the problems and acknowledges them. This links to a central feature of the work, perhaps best described by Levy (2004) as containment and validation – containment of the powerful internal states and anxieties and validation of the reality of the external trauma. The validation of current external realities that may impinge on the capacity to engage in the work is also an important part of the development of the therapeutic alliance.

Trauma-informed care and service user involvement

The development of principles of Trauma-informed Care has contributed to an understanding of the adaptations that may be required when working with traumatised individuals. These have been described in many different ways but at its core being trauma-informed requires a recognition of the need to work in ways which promote:

(1) Safety
(2) Trustworthiness and transparency
(3) Collaboration and mutuality
(4) Empowerment, voice and choice
(5) Peer support and mutual self-help
(6) The recognition of cultural, historic and gender issues.

With these principles in mind, we have set up a Trauma Service panel composed of a number of staff and current patients who work together to address a variety of practical issues within the service, such as looking at the written communication that is given to patients, as well as efforts at co-production. One example of this is that we were successful in bidding for a small amount of charities' money to set up a lending library of trauma-related literature for patients. This was co-produced with a small working group from the panel. We hope that this work will lead to the development of peer support groups within the service and in time to further co-production and co-delivery.

Phase two of the therapeutic journey will become possible when there is sufficient therapeutic alliance and capacity to manage the window of tolerance. For some patients this may be facilitated by the use of other modalities such as EMDR, trauma-focused CBT or Narrative Exposure Therapy (NET). In our experience, if a patient is distressed by re-experiencing phenomena such as nightmares, flashbacks, intrusive images or somatic sensations, these trauma focused interventions can be especially helpful. We have found that it is best done by the same therapist if feasible and incorporated into the therapy, rather than needing to introduce the modality through another therapist. Inevitably, this raises complex and interesting issues around the 'action' that one is taking and the propensity for action to become enactment. The reality of the need for action across the variety of interventions we offer necessitates a close examination through supervision and reflective spaces to attend to this tightrope we find ourselves on.

Whatever modality or way of working we are using, we bring our psychoanalytic understanding of what is happening in the room for consideration and thought. Indeed, we would see that in phase two, working with the transference is a trauma-focused therapy since the repetition compulsion will bring the traumatic scenario into the transference. Enactments, especially when one is working with paranoid-schizoid anxieties and projective identification is rife, are inevitable. They provide an understanding of the unconscious meanings and phantasies linked to the trauma and the ways in which these are being repeated through action within relationships.

The individual work, whether weekly or fortnightly, is conducted face to face rather than on the couch. We feel this is often important for a number of reasons. It generally facilitates a reduction in persecutory anxiety about the therapist and enables the patient to check on the state of mind of the therapist. It can facilitate activation of Porges' Ventral Vagus system of attachment, providing a sense of safety through the non-verbal interaction of the dyad. It facilitates the activation of mirror neurones so that a relaxed, engaged and curious stance in the therapist may be mirrored by the patient at an unconscious level. In these different ways, it allows the patient feedback on what is going on at a non-verbal level in the room between patient and therapist. I believe this links with what Schore (2009) is referring to when he describes the psycho-biologically attuned therapist acting as an interactive affect regulator of the patient who is dysregulated. He suggests that alongside the more traditional work of transference interpretation (linked to the left hemisphere of the brain), the therapeutic relationship needs to work in the implicit regulatory structures of the patient's and analyst's right brain.

For many patients with C-PTSD to even consider using a couch in a more traditional psychoanalytic setting would serve to highlight too painfully the inequality of the relationship and would suggest an authority and power imbalance in the therapeutic work that would feel reminiscent of power imbalances that led to traumatic experiences. Clearly, this issue goes far beyond the concrete nature of the setting and highlights a need to take a stance, which one may describe as 'working alongside'. This may be reflected in a more mutually collaborative working and may inform the style in which interpretations are offered. For instance, an interpretation that is couched in a 'You feel this' manner may be experienced as distancing, authoritarian and persecutory. This does not mean the therapist does not own her authority or recognize the reality of the power imbalance that is inherent in the therapeutic situation but rather that her style does not feel as though she is forcing the patient to be cognizant of this at all times.

Shame

Face-to-face work also has its difficulties, especially when there is considerable shame. Whilst some therapists are more able to keep a neutral expression than others, for many patients this neutrality can also be problematic as it creates a distance that may be experienced as being with an unfeeling or uninterested other. For other patients, to see the impact of their words on the therapist's face can stir up enormous anxiety of being overwhelming or damaging.

The ubiquity of shame, especially with historical (non-recent) sexual abuse has also been a driving factor for us setting up a specialist arm of the service for this group. The central therapeutic option here is to provide one-year groups – for women, for young women (under 30 years) and hopefully soon for men. The groups also serve to address understandable fears and anxieties that individual therapy can activate in relation to power dynamics and, although often provoking considerable anxiety, the group can offer a safe space to address the impact of these experiences.

Adapting to particular needs of different groups of patients has also led to a number of partnerships that have been developed with the voluntary sector. This includes a three-year partnership with a charity that offered a therapeutic community to homeless veterans whilst we offered individual trauma therapy. We have also had a long-running partnership with the British Red Cross (BRC) where a small group of honorary therapists worked alongside caseworkers in the Refugee and International Family Tracing Services in the BRC to offer therapeutic trauma consultations and therapy to asylum seekers.

Endings and new beginnings

We see the final phase of reconnection/reintegration as also including work on endings and the mourning that this entails. The grief that ending activates is inextricably linked to the mourning that has often not occurred in relation to the traumatic experiences. At the same time, the need to facilitate a connection with external realities, especially other relationships runs alongside this. One important new development for the service in this area has been setting up a trauma gardening group. This provides an opportunity for social connection in a safe setting as well as connection with nature and the importance of physical activity. In time, we also hope to see a peer support group that could support and provide a bridge during this transition as therapy ends.

Alongside this clinical work, the Tavistock Trauma Service offers consultation to organizations working with traumatised individuals or who have been traumatised themselves. This has included work with organizations linked to the London Bombings, the Grenfell Tower Fire and so on. As well as the Tavistock one-year trauma course and the regular external lectures on trauma, the service also offers a wide variety of trainings and events nationally and internationally.

Conclusion

The Trauma Service is indebted to a small group of highly motivated and committed staff members who demonstrate creativity and a willingness to develop innovative ways of working whilst holding their analytic frame. It could also not function without the generosity and skill of honorary therapists, linking perhaps to the beginnings of the Tavistock when before the NHS, all staff worked in a voluntary capacity. The realities of limited resources, greater and growing demand and need, and the pressures within the NHS setting to offer brief interventions are a constant threat to the service and its survival. We see in the broader socio-political settings evidence of so much ongoing trauma including the impact of the Covid pandemic, the Black Lives Matter Movement, the Climate Emergency, Men's Violence towards Women to name but a few. There is a growing need to address the impact of trauma within mental health services and more broadly within communities, and we hope that the work of the service will survive and continue to address these needs into the future.

Acknowledgements

This paper would not have been possible without the staff, trainees and honorary therapists of the Tavistock Trauma Service and without the patients in the service. Thanks are also due to Graham Music, who allowed me the honour of sharing a platform with him to give the centenary lecture.

Disclosure statement

No potential conflict of interest was reported by the author(s).

References

Allen, J. G. (2001). *Traumatic relationships and serious mental disorders*. Wiley.

Bion, W. R. (1963). *Elements of psychoanalysis*. William Heinemann, Medical Books. (Reprinted London: Karnac Books, 1984).

Bollas, C. (1987). *The shadow of the object: Psychoanalysis of the unthought known*. Columbia University Press.

Cloitre, M., Courtois, C. A., Charuvastra, A., Carapezza, R., Stolbach, B. C., & Green, B. L. (2011). Treatment of complex PTSD: Results of the ISTSS expert clinician survey on best practices. *Journal of Traumatic Stress*, *24*(6), 615–627. https://doi.org/10.1002/jts.20697

Cloitre, M., Courtois, C. A., Ford, J. D., Green, B. L., Alexander, P., Briere, J., Herman, J., Lanius, R., Pearlman, L., Stolbach, J., van der Kolk, B., & van der Hart, O. (2012). *The ISTSS expert consensus treatment guidelines for complex PTSD in adults*. International Society of Traumatic Stress Studies.

Cloitre, M., Garvert, D. W., Weiss, B., Carlson, E. B., & Bryant, R. A. (2014). Distinguishing PTSD, complex PTSD, and borderline personality disorder: A latent class analysis. *European Journal of Psychotraumatology*, *5*(1), 25097. https://doi.org/10.3402/ejpt.v5.25097

Fonagy, P., Gergely, G., Jurist, E., & Target, M. (2002). *Affect regulation mentalization and the development of the self*. Other Press.

Freud, S. (1920). *Beyond the pleasure principle, S.E.18*. Hogarth.

Garland, C. (Ed). (1998). *Understanding trauma: A psychoanalytic approach*. Tavistock Book Series.

Heimann, P. (1950). On countertransference. *International Journal of Psychoanalysis*, *31*, 81–84.

Herman, J. L. (1992). Complex PTSD: A syndrome in survivors of prolonged and repeated trauma. *Journal of Traumatic Stress*, *5*(3), 377–391. https://doi.org/10.1002/jts.2490050305

Holinger, P. C. (1999). Non-interpretative intervention in psychoanalysis and psychotherapy: A developmental perspective. *Psychoanalytic Psychology*, *16*(2), 233–253. https://doi.org/10.1037/0736-9735.16.2.233

Johnstone, L., & Boyle, M. (2018). The power threat meaning framework: An alternative nondiagnostic conceptual system. *Journal of Humanistic Psychology*. Advance online publication. https://doi.org/10.1177/0022167818793289.

Joseph, B. (1985). Transference: The total situation. *International Journal of Psychoanalysis*, *66* (4) , 447–454.

Joseph, B. (1992). Psychic Change: Some Perspectives. *International Journal of Psychoanalysis*, *73* (2) , 237–243.

Klein, M. (1946). Notes on some schizoid mechanisms. *International Journal of Psychoanalysis*, *27*, 99–110.

Levy, S. (2004). Containment and Validation. In S. Levy, and A. Lemma (Eds.), *The perversion of loss: Psychoanalytic reflections on trauma* (pp. 50-70). Whurr Publishers .

Liotti, G. (2011). Attachment disorganization and the clinical dialogue: Theme and variations. In J. Solomon, and C. George (Eds.), *Disorganisation of attachment and caregiving* (pp. 383–413). Guildford Press.

Luyten, P., Campbell, C., & Fonagy, P. (2019). Borderline personality disorder, complex trauma, and problems with self and identity: A social-communicative approach. *Journal of Personality*, *88*(Feb), 88–105. https://doi.org/10.1111/jopy.12483

Lyons-Ruth, K. (2001). The two-person construction of defences: Disorganized attachment strategies, unintegrated mental states and hostile/helpless relational processes. *Psychologist Psychoanalyst*, *21*(1), 40–45. https://doi.org/10.1080/15289168.2002.10486422.

Mackin, D., Kotov, R., Perlman, G., Nelson, B., Goldstein, B., Hajcak, G., & Klein, D. (2019). Reward processing and future life stress: Stress generation pathway to depression. *Journal of Abnormal Psychology*, *128*(4), 305–314. https://doi.org/10.1037/abn0000427

Main, M., & Solomon, J. (1990). Procedures for identifying infants as disorganized/ disoriented during the Ainsworth strange situation. In M. T. Greenberg (Ed.), *Attachment in the preschool years: Theory, research and intervention* (pp. 121–160). The University of Chicago Press.

National Institute for Clinical Excellence. (2019). *Post-traumatic Stress Disorder: The management of PTSD in adults and children in primary and secondary care*. Gaskell.

Porges, S. W. (2011). *The polyvagal theory: Neurophysiological foundations of emotions, attachment, communication and self-regulation*. Norton.

Schore, A. N. (2009). Attachment trauma and the developing right brain: Origins of pathological dissociation. In P. F. Dell & J. F. O'Neil (Eds.), *Dissociation and the dissociative disorders: DSM-V and beyond* (pp. 107–141). Routledge.

Segal, H. (1957). Notes on symbol formation. *International Journal of Psychoanalysis*, *38*, 391–405.

Siegel, D. J. (1999). *The developing mind: How relationships and the brain interact to shape who we are*. Guilford Press.

Stern, D. B. (1997). *Unformulated experience: From dissociation to imagination in psychoanalysis*. Analytic Press.

Taylor, S. E., Klein, L. C., Lewis, B. P., Gruenewald, T. L., Gurung, R. A. R., & Updegraff, J. A. (2000). Biobehavioural responses to stress in females: Tend-and-befriend. Not fight-or-flight. *Psychological Review*, *107*(3), 411–429. https://doi.org/10.1037/0033-295X.107.3.411

Tottenham, N., Hare, T. A., Millner, A., Gilhooly, T., Zevin, J. D., & Casey, B. J. (2011). Elevated amygdala response to faces following early deprivation. *Developmental Science*, *14*(2), 190–204. https://doi.org/10.1111/j.1467-7687.2010.00971.x

Van der Kolk, B. (2014). *The body keeps the score: Brain, mind, and body in the healing of trauma*. Penguin.

Being safe and being brave: new thoughts on trauma, and adaptations to technique

Graham Music

This paper outlines ways in which more traditional psychoanalytic technique has been challenged by new findings about trauma and the optimal ways in which it can be worked with. In particular it outlines how therapists need to become much more knowledgeable about the risks of retriggering PTSD symptoms, and about dissociative symptomatology. In addition, in some cases it is suggested that psychoanalytic therapists might become braver in helping victims of trauma to feel anger about what happened to them, and that often for optimal recovery anger and rage needs to precede remorse, reparation and a bearing of depressive anxieties

Introduction: trauma as a challenge

Current psychoanalytic technique has been challenged by new knowledge about trauma. Psychoanalysis has an honourable early tradition of working with trauma (e.g., Ferenczi, 1926), as well as of awareness of the body (Reich, 1945), and in recent decades psychoanalytic thinking about trauma has been revived in work with adults (e.g., Garland, 2018) and children (e.g., Kenrick et al., 2006; Lanyado, 2003; Music, 2019). However I suggest that there are distinct ways in which our therapeutic technique can be enhanced by scientific understandings of trauma, including neurobiology.

In the first section of the paper, I show how a lack of understanding of trauma and dissociation can lead to a danger of therapeutic failure by precipitating re-traumatisation. I suggest that we learn how to recognise dissociative states, how to work with bodily manifestations of trauma, and importantly, learn that successful work with trauma means initially avoiding focus on the deepest anxieties, and hence ensuring there is no retriggering of trauma.

In the second half of the paper, I suggest that recent psychoanalytic technique has sometimes played too much heed to enabling people to move into depressive anxieties, to manage reparation, guilt and sadness, and in that process we can undermine the healing that can occur when anger, rage and courage can be owned as developmentally helpful and not defensive.

Trauma and dissociation

Trauma is overwhelming, sometimes life threatening, and often leads to survival responses of numbing and quietening, and out of body states. In trauma people can literally become 'thoughtless', go into a stupor (stupefaction) and become speechless. This is an understandable response when faced with a life-threatening event, such as being attacked by a predator. The people who suffer the most worrying symptoms have had not just one such experience but rather multiple early traumas (Van der Kolk, 2017). If someone has consistently been exposed to terrifying events, such as being tortured, witnessing or being the victim of constant violence, or being sexually abused, recovery will be much harder and they will spend a lot of time in or on the verge of such shutdown states.

Such trauma leaves people feeling unsafe to the core of their beings and needing specific kinds of help. If I have been multiply traumatised and am in a dissociated shut-down state, I will struggle, for example, to experience strong feelings, to face memories, or even to respond to playfulness and empathy. Indeed, the very idea of starting to feel feelings can provoke anxiety and fear. Feeling feelings often means re-experiencing terrifying trauma symptoms that dissociative processes are designed to help trauma victims not to feel.

For good reason many newer forms of trauma therapy, such as Compassion Focussed Therapy (Gilbert, 2019) Sensorimotor therapy (Ogden, 2006) or EMDR (Parnell, 2013), expend much effort building up what they call resources, inner states that feel safe, easeful and self-caring. Such ideas, and in particular the need to actively help people feel safe, have not been part of traditional psychoanalytic technique. In trauma it is vital to turn off the body's hyperalert danger signals, to reset and reboot somatic and psychological systems by facilitating a sense of safeness, without which pain and trauma cannot be processed. Some version of this needs to be incorporated into psychoanalytically informed work with trauma.

Early mistakes. Barak

For many years I did not understand trauma and its effects. Consequently, I made many mistakes, and my well-intentioned if naïve approach was common when I started out. Some decades ago, I saw a young man who I call Barak. He was walking in a local park with his girlfriend when they experienced a violent racially motivated attack. She was sexually assaulted, and he was pinned down and had to watch, feeling helpless. Eventually she broke free and ran, but he was badly beaten.

On meeting he seemed appropriately nervous if somewhat edgy. I had been trained to naively expect that he, like most, would be glad of the opportunity to talk about and process the incident, that this would bring relief. In fact, the opposite transpired. When I asked about what happened, he became agitated, moving his body jerkily, as if having tics, sweat appearing on his brow, his eyes faraway.

I found myself holding my breath anxiously, and I felt cold, my mind seemingly shutting down, something I have since experienced often with traumatised patients.

It is worth imagining what Barak experienced. The beating he had received was extremely severe, leaving him with broken bones and in terrible pain, but worse, he had also been powerless to help his girlfriend. He in fact remembered little of the incident, had gone into the kind of numbed state, sometimes wrongly called the freeze response, an ancient defence mechanism in the face of life-threat and overwhelming pain. We numb down, literally having an analgesic opioid response which stops pain, breathing becoming shallow and heart rate lowering dramatically, a response called bradycardia. We might even feel as if we have left our body, and indeed sexual abuse victims often describe watching the abuse from above.

This is shut-down much like that seen in what Naviaux (2020) calls the cell-danger response. Body temperature reduces, vocalisation stops, and we see tonic immobilisation, a kind of paralysis. Other symptoms include pupils dilating and sweating. Of course, looking dead enhances the chances of survival as most predators will not risk eating something that might be toxic.

Just before such extreme responses is when we are likely to see freeze, which in fact is a more alert state. In freeze we are preparing, sometimes bracing, and the options of either fight or flight remain. In freeze we are immobile, heart rate lowered (Fragkaki et al., 2017), but probably orienting, scanning the environment, non-consciously taking in any signs of immediate danger, preparing to actively make oneself safe. If this fails, we move to the next stage, from freezing to tonic immobility.

All this is relevant to Barak. Being confronted by four large youths with clubs, he realised he could not fight back, or even run, so he was left helpless, with only the last resort strategies of numbing or flopping available to him. In fleeing, one retains some control, it is energising and requires activity, agency, and hope, fighting even more so. Barak did not have these options.

When I naively asked Barak about what had happened, he became agitated but then withdrawn, shut away. His gait was robotic, he seemed almost ghostly in his lack of presence, showing signs of moving into what is sometimes called catalepsy, an immobility often seen in trauma and related to that seen in catatonic states. He struggled to speak but with careful questioning I discovered that when I had asked questions about the attack, he had experienced flashbacks. He admitted he was often assailed by these, leaving him feeling unsafe about even leaving his home.

Thus, such numbing is a sensible adaptation but comes at a cost. His very slow heart rate, numbing down, acting submissive or ‘dead’, were helpful defence mechanisms. His dissociation was also helpful, freeing him from overwhelming thoughts and feelings which otherwise meant re-experiencing terror. His body and nervous system still believed the threat was present and this was not going to be changed by a naïve therapist suggesting that it is helpful to talk about his trauma.

My lack of early training in trauma meant I knew little about flashbacks, dissociation, or states such as depersonalisation or derealisation. I was out of my depth. Barak did not continue with therapy and voted with his feet, probably making the right decision. I would approach his case very differently today.

For him, life and liveliness were terrifying, memories were traumatising, empathy made no sense and what Barak needed more than anything, at least initially was a sense of feeling safe, something he had little experience of. His body and being was in cell-danger response and he needed to be held in a softer, almost cotton-wool container where he could be helped to have his nervous system recalibrated, to reboot and reset.

Barak was a mixture of too floppy and too tense with very little in between. His movement lacked grace and ease, he was constantly vigilant and expecting danger. His breathing was shallow, he felt little ease, and any energy was in the service of turning away and self-protection, closing down not turning towards experience and hope. This was all appropriate and understandable given his early experiences. I now suggest how we can help such people in dissociated shut-down states begin to come back into life again.

Rana part 1: immobilisation for safety

Rana came to see me in her early 30s after falling in love with someone who had shown no interest in her. She had had a tough life, shunted between foster homes as a child, never consistently cared for or held in mind, moving from town to town and school to school, and experiencing a childhood of parental neglect and being bullied in school.

She clearly needed and wanted my help but not surprisingly was as distrustful of me as she was of most people. She had never been in a relationship, had very few friends and lived an isolated life, working in an unchallenging administrative role and returning to a solitary flat. Fear leads to shut down which leads to disconnection, and a withdrawn hopelessness, as we have seen. I was struck by the floppiness in her body which could be mistaken for calmness. Therapy was a challenge as she had developed a personality around avoiding being seen, not revealing herself, staying under the radar.

Rana was exposed to inappropriate males as a child, and might have been sexually abused, but she had no memory of this. This was possibly when she first went into extreme 'flop' immobile postures, although this could have also happened due to early neglect. Multiple factors can give rise to such a presentation. At school she would hide in a corner of the playground clinging to a book, hair over her face and hoodie over her head, for fear of the next bullying episode. This is a classic shut-down response to trauma. Like all mammals, when serious danger is present, humans will become still, 'playing possum', as this aids chances of survival.

As the infamous psychiatrist R.D. Laing in *The Divided Self* wrote (Laing, 1969) 'In a world full of danger, to be a potentially see-able object is to be constantly exposed to danger. . . . The obvious defence against such a danger is to make oneself invisible in one way or another.' Of course, being visible exposes one to potential attacks by predators, and the school playground was a frightening danger-zone for Rana.

Decades after the serious trauma, she was still living in a nightmare world of fear and constant danger signals. It was easy to mistake her stillness for being relaxed, an all-too-common error. When people do not obviously act stressed, they can be misperceived as 'calm', even 'cool'. There is some truth in this. The point of such shutting down is not just to be unseen, but also to not feel what is too difficult to feel. She was barely conscious of her bodily stillness, or of the shallowness of her breath and inexpressiveness of her face. These danger responses had once served her well but now kept her from living an emotionally rich life. She needed a reset and reboot.

Rana needed help initially to feel safer in her body and I was more active in my facilitation of body awareness than I would once have been. One of the first things I focused on was her breathing. Rather than suggesting she breath more deeply I first asked what her breath felt like. 'I can't really feel it' she replied. I asked her to put her hand on her chest and feel any movement. I then asked if it felt safe to loosen or deepen her breath a tiny bit and what that felt like. She did this and said it felt scary, it made her nervous. Breathing deeply requires some trust that the world feels safe, that there is no immediate danger. I suggested instead that she really breathed in, as if very tense, and tighten up her breath as if she were in real danger, 'lets get to know what it feels like to really hold your breath'. She did this and then said, 'I realise how constricted I am feeling, I had never noticed'. The first tears I had seen seeped into her eyes.

This was a slow incremental process, trying out a deeper breath, seeing how it felt, then ensuring she felt safe enough to return to her comfort zone. As I often find, memories, thoughts and feelings flooded into the session, and we had to go carefully. Ease and trusting in safeness feel risky when our minds and bodies are signalling ever-present danger.

Some weeks later I asked her to widen her shoulders, allow a breath into her belly and let her chest (heart) open. Tears streamed down her face. She had remembered some good feelings, times with a foster carer who had loved and protected her. The image of this kind woman became a symbol of self-compassion, an inner voice she could turn to for support, who could help her trust in this new sense of safeness. She had that bitter-sweet feeling of knowing that opening up to hope felt good but still wanting to fight it, feeling the urge to shut-down again, back to what she knew all too well.

We began to explore what it felt like to be seen and noticed, by a male colleague at work, by me, another man, and the mixed feelings this evoked. She came to sessions with stories of what she was now noticing, such as how quickly she closed up like a clam when someone looked at her, or how she tensed up when she had an anxious thought. Becoming able to notice herself tighten up allowed her to then let go, something mindfulness also teaches us, allowing the tension and watching it from a more capacious containing place, almost cradling the tension, rather than immediately acting on the temptation to close or self-protect.

Much of the initial work with Rana was in such resetting, safening, helping danger signals lessen and trusting a new sense of hope. Could she look around and feel safe and not tense up? Could she look someone in the eye and not be scared? Could she catch herself tensing and help herself by, for example, watching her breath? The first stage of coming back into life for Rana was allowing a pulsing in her being, in the breath, in the sensations in her body, an aliveness she had long needed to close down against.

Sometimes this brought up memories, such as of a girl who bullied her. I never sought out those memories, but when they arose, we worked carefully with them. The challenge is to ensure we do not re-traumatise, not re-signal danger, but to tiptoe up to trauma, gently be with it and move back to safety, and repeat the process time and again. Safeness is the foundation for both building the equipment to process and metabolise feelings, and then for sparking into life.

Her subdued lacklustre floppiness started to shapeshift into more toned muscularity, to healthy tension. Her beliefs that 'I must stay still otherwise it is too dangerous', or 'it is safer to withdraw', were being challenged. Her inertia had come from paralysing fear but slowly she could soften, open, and feel more trust, and in time even feel rage and fury at what happened to her. This bred life, heat, strength, and courage, indeed spark, an energetic current that could be powerful. We will meet her again and hear more about such post-safening developments later in the paper.

Not feeling real

Rana was shut down but less dissociated than Mendy, a late adolescent by the time I met him. Mendy had suffered even more severe trauma, including serious physical and sexual violence at home. As with many inert, lifeless almost de-sparked people, he had few friends at school, struggled to interact with anyone and had managed adolescence by retreating to computer games, pornography and fugue-like numbed states.

When I met him, he seemed lifeless, and had given up hope that anyone might understand how awful he felt. He was not only feelingless, in a semi-catatonic way, but for much of his life he felt unreal, not really present. His numbness had helped stave off earlier unbearable terror and turmoil, but this had shrivelled his emotional processing capacities, and now he had little life-force available, and his priors were all of danger and fear.

Mendy was another who reported that when he was being beaten, and sexually assaulted as a child he had a literal experience of floating above his body watching the abuse, a classic dissociation from unbearable experiences. The gain was that he did not have to experience the trauma, but the loss was that in such states he felt numb, disembodied and not real.

Feeling unreal in dissociation commonly takes two forms, often seen as one syndrome, called DPDR, meaning depersonalisation and derealisation. In depersonalisation (DP) you feel as if you are detached from yourself, as if watching yourself from the outside, like in a movie. This is perhaps why the Truman Show struck such a nerve for so many people. In depersonalisation people are out of touch with body sensations, often unable to feel emotions, can feel robotic, and their mind can feel 'fuggy', as if wrapped in cotton wool.

Derealisation (DR) is similar but here the external world and sometimes other people do not feel quite real. Mendy described watching events and people as if through a veil, or a glass wall. Sometimes sufferers have a heightened awareness of their surroundings, with distorted sense of how large or small, near or far, objects are. Possibly this helps in traumatic events; if someone comes at you with a knife you will be hyperaware of that knife, it will loom very large but other objects will not. Yet paradoxically things can also feel blurry and colourless. This possibly comes with the need for distance from experiences and to take the emotional tone and hue out.

Mendy was sometimes so shutdown that he looked barely conscious. At best he had a compliant wan smile, far from a lively genuine 'Duchenne' smile. Teachers would get frustrated, and he would be targeted for being stubborn, refusing to concentrate, and teased for being boring. Mendy often was 'spaced-out' and when with him, I felt spacey too, not fully present. Probably not feeling his own bodily presence was a necessary way of protecting himself when he was being beaten to an inch of his life by his father. However, he knew his current state was not normal, and he hated it, felt powerless and worried about his mental health.

Working with DPDR is difficult, in part because sufferers feel so hopeless and this gets transmitted to those around them, including friends, family and therapists. DPDR is not something you can change just by trying harder. One cannot try to feel real! Change is slow and incremental and follows what we might call an order of operations. As with Rana, Mendy needed first of all to feel safe, we needed to turn down the danger signals, not easy given the extent of the violence he had suffered. Symptoms that develop to protect a trauma sufferer will not be let go of easily. We have to be nervous system whisperers who help an over-alert nervous system believe that there is no longer real danger. Only then can there be a quieting, and of a kind that is known in one's body, not by cognitive persuasion or efforting, but deep down, almost at a cellular level.

The environments of sufferers, whether their living and working environments or a therapy space, need to feel as safe as possible, otherwise positive change can easily get undone. With Mendy I started with a classic activity, orienting, or in other words, checking out the space, carefully looking around the room with me supporting him. Orienting is something we often see in an initial freeze reaction and is a kind of response preparation, one in which heart rate tends to come down, orienting giving some sense of control and potential for decision-making.

From here we could move onto helping him feel safer in his body. There are multiple ways this can happen, no rulebook, each person being different. I often start with deepening the breath. With Mendy this did not work and only increased his panic. I used other techniques such as trying to imagine a time and space when he had felt safe and getting to know the accompanying feelings of safeness in his body, such as of more relaxed muscles. He remembered a kindly female neighbour who gave him respite from being beaten. I asked him to recall what being with her had felt like, what his body remembered about the safeness she provided, what he felt when she showed kindness or curiosity. For some people, Mendy included, it is like building new memories from scratch, as they have had so little real experience of feeling safe. Many find imagining or building such a compassionate figure helpful, whether a person they knew, a religious figure, or even a loved pet.

Although Mendy became triggered if I worked with his breath, I could slowly help him be in touch with basic body sensations, such as the feeling of his feet on the floor or his bottom on a chair, the feelings in his fingers or toes, the pulsing of blood flow, an awareness of aches and pains, or the sensation of the breath moving in his chest. These are ways of grounding and learning to be more present and safer. We had to go cautiously because for Mendy and many others, it had felt dangerous to even feel physical sensations.

Once a feeling of safeness begins to be built other changes can follow, such as deeper breathing, moments of relaxation, an increased sense of trust. Until this happens there is no possibility of building a container to process trauma. Increasing trust and ease must come first, starting with a safe experiencing of body sensation. I often liken this to the experience of one's fingers thawing out after being frozen. It can tingle and hurt, we might resist it, but we know it will be for the best in the end. With unfreezing from trauma, the process needs to be very gradual.

Mendy slowly made use of these interventions, and by the end could go out into the world, to shops or places of work, and find ways of managing feeling triggered. For example, when he realised he was triggered, he could now note that his breath was quickening and chest tightening, and slowly re-regulate himself, by for example, feeling his feet on the floor, and watching other body sensations. It was his increasing ability to be aware of his body which was the real turning point. Watching his sensations, his muscles tensing, noticing when he wanted to flee, enabled the slow thawing of his DPDR symptoms. He could be more present with his experiences, his memories of trauma for example, which could be stayed with as we stayed with the accompanying body sensations. This newfound bodily awareness also gave him confidence that he could go out into the world safely, with more hope, less fear and contraction, and increased faith that he could feel safe, and in time, be an active participant in life.

Ripe for anger and protest

Trauma can kill off spark, energy, what Freud called *libido*, or lifeforce. For some, that spark has never developed, while for others it was repressed or deactivated, or has become blocked, and needs freeing or loosening up. Early psychoanalysts, including the early Freud knew this, as did followers such as Reich (1945) and Ferenczi (1926), and asserted the importance of freeing up frozen energy, often frozen protest.

We can think of this kind of shut-down is seen in learned helplessness, as researched by Seligman (Maier & Seligman, 1976). In rather cruel experiments dogs were given electric shocks. Some dogs could stop these by pressing a lever while others had no such opportunity. The dogs lacking any control would no longer try to escape even when it was possible to do so. In effect their 'learnt helplessness' became a kind of character trait, the animals looking fearful and hopeless and showing symptoms very like human depression and anxiety. They, and many people I have worked with, might be described as having had their spirits broken by both fear and a lack of control over their fate.

The psychiatrist Viktor Frankel, himself an Auschwitz inmate, reported how concentration camp survivors, when liberated, initially walked out of the camp gates, but then returned to lie down within the camp borders. They could not believe that freedom was really safe to reach for. This is what we see in many traumatised people who often do not protest against violence, or abuse, and take on a given-up or hopeless stance, and this includes children and also adults who have been victims of sexual, domestic, or racial violence and are too accepting of their lot.

We repress and deny thoughts and feelings out of anxiety, fear, or guilt, but doing so comes at costs, such as feeling less alive. Learned helplessness is quashing of life, a trauma-induced fear resulting in a kind of paralysis which remains well after the perpetrator is gone. This is seen in people's bodies, such as in slumped hunched poses, heads bowed, and fearing to stand tall.

Most children of course cannot afford to get cross with or criticise their parents and so any blame or fault tends to be directed inwards, back at themselves, which is what I have seen in countless children from abusive backgrounds. This was beautifully described long ago by Fairbairn (1962) as the moral defence, in which it feels safer to be bad in a world ruled by a good god, than to be good in a world ruled by the devil.

Psychotherapists work hard to help people to mourn, grieve, manage sadness, allow vulnerability. These are all immensely important but for the kinds of states I describe here, something more active and energising is needed. In particular, rage and anger are appropriate responses to abuse and trauma and should not be bypassed.

If my father hits me, or my partner slaps me, it can be healthy to fight back, to feel strength instead of retreating into helplessness and given-upness. However, anger can be scary, we might fear being hit again, or alienate someone we feel we need. When asked how they feel about bad things that have happened to them, many say things like 'perhaps I deserved to be hit', or 'I should not have done that' or 'but I know he loves me really'. In psychoanalytic parlance, these are defensive forms of rationalisation.

Such rationalisation is seen when we move away from feelings into thoughts, a movement that often happens because feelings such as rage are scary. The fear that leads to learned helplessness can often lead to such defensive manoeuvres. But what is needed, instead, is help in getting closer to righteous anger, rage, and protest, really knowing and owning such feelings, in one's body, and in the depths of ones being. This enables people to become less fearful, and more able to believe that they can become powerful, strong, and energised.

Rana part 2. Rage and striated muscle

Rana, who I described earlier, was one such person. Neglected and bullied at school, abused by her parents and again in foster care, she had little confidence, and her body was floppy and lifeless. I often felt that I could almost blow her over, as if she had given away all her power. We had already worked hard on developing a sense of security and after a long period of work focusing on this, she could now sooth herself when she was anxious, by various mechanisms which she used to comforted herself when she was feeling triggered.

With this development of her new sense of security, we could begin to look at the more difficult feelings. Her floppiness, hunched pose and lack of energy were all signs of a depressed hopelessness, an embodied belief that danger was still constantly lurking, and she was powerless against it. When we began to think about what happened to her, such as the bullying, she quickly went into rationalisations such as 'well it's all in the past now', or worse 'but I feel I am just a monster'. At one point, her new boss was treating her in a way that was clearly unfair, yet she could not really see this. If I asked her how she felt towards her boss for what he did and she said, 'well I did make a mistake, I am always getting things wrong'. Digging a bit deeper we found depths of shame and self-contempt written into her body, gestures, voice and probably deep into her brain and cells.

Slowly she began to see what she was doing to herself, and what she was not doing for herself. I picked up on how self-deprecating she was with me, and how overly forgiving she was when I got something wrong. 'Oh but you did not mean it' she would say. She was hugely invested in being 'nice', but this was a placatory niceness. For her, others needed to be 'kept sweet' or else they might hurt her.

I suggested she try to imagine what it might feel like to be angry. She had never had the relief one feels when someone accepts one's anger and is not destroyed by it, but rather remains steadfastly there, strong and present, and non-retaliatory. As Winnicott helped us understand (Winnicott, 1971), having one's rage heard and survived without retaliation gives a perception that one's feelings are not dangerous and leads to a sense of having a separate self, not always having to tiptoe around minefields. This is energising, sparking and also facilitates an opening up to emotional connection rather than the closing down we see when danger signals are high.

Slowly Rana began to be able to stand up for herself more. At work she challenged her boss, becoming less likely to take criticism 'lying down'. We role-played interactions in which she began to learn what it feels like to 'stand up' for herself, to 'hold her head up high' and 'look the other in the eye', rather than be submissive. This began to translate into other areas of her life. She started not to apologise, no longer saying 'sorry to ask you', or 'I hope you don't mind', but instead beginning to feel that she had a right to ask for things. Her over-zealous worry that those around her might be upset, including me, began to abate and instead she became more assertive.

Her body seemed to be changing, she had energy in her limbs, colour was coming to her cheeks, her chest and heart area were opening, her head held up, she moved with confidence, even determination, with much less hint of apology or deference. I noted this and asked what else had changed and to my amazement, she told me that she was no longer just doing gentle 'yin' yoga but had started a more active form which contain 'warrior' poses, and she had even begun doing some strength training. Some muscularity was growing, in both mind and body, and she also had begun to look much more attractive. Men were noticing her on the street, and although this was unnerving, she was developing a new kind of confidence.

This was not a straightforward process; the gains came with a cost. We had to find the courage to become assertive, to feel anger and rage, to change deep patterns and priors. When her boss had preferentially privileged a colleague over her, I asked, 'So what do you want to say to him?'. 'Well, he was not being very nice'. 'Okay', I would reply, 'but that is not how you feel, so how do you feel towards him for what he did?'. Well, she might say, 'I have got used to it now'. I pushed more, 'Hmm, again that is not saying what you feel. I notice how your jaw is clenched and your fist tensed, what would they like to do?'. 'Oh nothing' she said a bit shamefaced as she tried to let go of the tension. I clenched my own fists and said forcefully 'I do that when I am really angry, sometimes it feels good to be angry'.

She looked interested and breathed more deeply, but soon went back to a more passive stance. Her default position was to be compliant, and she had justified this with a kind of moral superiority, believing that anger and aggression were bad, that being forceful is not 'nice'. This though came at a huge cost. I challenged her again and she was able, with prompting, to raise her head and say forcefully how angry she was. I asked her to stand up and express the feelings, imagining her boss in front of her. As she did this the energy in her body changed, she was leaning forward, and showed real power. Afterwards we carefully debriefed. I asked how she felt. She was breathing deeply now, looking proud, and definitely energised. A bit later tears came, partly of relief, and also a genuine sadness and compassion for the Rana who had always suffered by not daring to take herself seriously.

This aspect of the work owed much to a psychoanalytically informed model of therapy called ISTDP (Intensive Short Term Dynamic Psychotherapy), rooted in the work of Malan at the Tavistock Clinic (Malan, 1976), and developed later by Davanloo (1979). ISTDP has an understanding of body states, trauma and attachment. In its technique it distinguishes between a readiness to embrace feelings such as anger, observable in straited muscle tension, as opposed to the more dissociative responses seen in smooth muscle presentations. This thinking has been taken forward and researched impressively by Abbass (2015) and others.

Rana's clenched fists and jaw were classic signs of 'striated' muscle tone, the kind which shows there is energy and tension which is ready to be brought out and expressed. Sometimes when I pushed Rana too far, or said something that was too much to bear, she would retreat into physiological states which are the opposite, into energyless 'smooth muscle' states. For Rana this could be a stomach cramp, or feeling faint, or a headache. Smooth muscle presentations can also include symptoms such as irritable bowel syndrome, migraines, nausea, diarrhoea, the need to suddenly urinate, back pain, amongst others. Physiologically smooth muscles are in the digestive tract and blood vessels, and out of conscious control. When a feeling, like rage or upset is too much to bear then smooth muscle presentations often result.

We can think of smooth muscle defences as a way of avoiding or repressing strong feelings which cannot be owned or faced. By developing a sufficiently capacious container to allow, feel and express repressed feelings we develop more energy, spark, and a capacity for connecting rather than closing down. In Rana, we saw movement towards, not away, from life, more healthy muscularity, a freeing of energy, genuine sparking. One of the most exciting things about freeing up such damned-up energy is that many physiological symptoms, too often termed psychosomatic, simply fade away. If we can express our rage and anger, for example, and do not need to repress or deny these feelings, then research shows that physiological symptoms common in smooth muscle states decrease (Abbass, 2015).

In dissociation such as smooth muscle states and cognitive dissonance, challenging defences is the last thing needed. Instead, the task is to prioritise restabilising, as with Rana initially, to reduce anxiety by facilitating physiological and psychological safeness, such as by returning to gentle body-based mindfulness exercises which helped her come out of numbed states. It is only when someone feels safe enough that striated muscle signals come online, and that is when one can challenge defences against pushed-away feelings and facilitate a freeing up of energy and lifeforce. The clues are in the body. In Rana's case, the fist clenching and jaw tightening were typical signs of muscular tension indicating that she was near being able to bear and express her rage.

Khenan

Hopefully, these ideas will become clear in meeting Khenan, a mixed-race young man from a complex background. He too had been bullied at school, subjected to racial abuse, after childhood experiences of being verbally attacked and hit by his stepfather, the father of his two younger siblings. He was a sad young man when I met him, nervous, unconfident, and awkward, getting through life with a false grin and keeping out of people's way. Although not slumped, he had a lack of solidity, of what Amy Cuddy called 'presence' (Cuddy, 2015), with a poor sense of himself and his worth.

He could not look people in the eye, had an elusive quality, always seeming about to retreat, suggesting that other people were not to be trusted. He carried deep pain and sadness near the surface, and further hidden away, was rage. In private he could spend hours staring into space or at computer games. He also complained of many physiological symptoms of the kind we often see with smooth muscle defences and unprocessed denied emotion, such as feeling nauseous, having back pain and headaches.

Such issues often become more complex when race enters the picture, possibly even more so for young black men. Khenan wanted to be cool, as well as strong and tough, the aspirations of his peer group. He was liked by teachers, but his academic potential was never taken seriously. Perhaps typical of black youth, he was encouraged in sports, and when he demonstrated a quicksilver ability on the football field, the bullying stopped and he could stay even more under the radar, with his big smile, gliding around the dangers of group-life, friendships, and adolescence, rather like he glided past tackles on the football pitch. I personally empathised, as being good at football and other sports had probably saved me from an awful adolescence and brought me some sense of self-worth.

Yet in truth, Khenan was very unhappy, often on the edge of imploding, or exploding, barely managing the powerful feelings that were taking him over. His overt reason for coming to therapy at 16-years-old was a painful experience of unrequited love leading to desperate, near suicidal feelings. Khenan had reluctantly had to admit to himself that he was gay, certainly not something he embraced, and given the homophobic adolescent culture he inhabited, this increased his sense of inadequacy.

Initially when we met, he seemed too ashamed to look at me, and I barely made out his face beneath his hoodie and scarves. When I asked about his sexual life, he looked excruciatingly awkward and then went into a kind of fugue state, his mind going numb and seeming almost not to be in the room with me. Later he explained that at such moments he wanted the earth to open up and swallow him.

At such moments he could barely string a sentence together, and such incoherence is typical of the cognitive dissonance often seen in emotional overload. This links with what happens in trauma, where broca's region in the brain, needed for speech, can go offline. As with Rana, the initial work was about developing a sense of safeness, helping him feel at ease in his body and trying to challenge his shame and self-hatred, about his sexuality and other areas. This included noting his self-effacing postures and how he moved overly cautiously and gingerly. Once an alliance and shared language was built, then his defences could slowly be challenged.

As he relaxed, colour came to his face, his breathing deepened, and he moved with more purpose. I began to see hopeful signs of striated muscle tension. I noted a look of disgust on his face when he described an interchange and I asked him to exaggerate the gesture and expand on it. For the first time I saw anger and some incipient power, suddenly there was a young man with strong feelings in the room, his disgust moving into rage. There was still a lot of fudging, intellectualising, shifting directions and I often felt like a spear-hunting fisherman trying to pin down my prey. This is very common. It is hard to get the balance between going in too hard, which can lead to smooth muscle and dissociative defences, and going too softly and cautiously, which can mean that feelings that are ready to be faced are avoided, leaving old symptoms and defences in place.

Real vitality requires energy and power, and defences against feelings like rage or grief can dampen our vitalising potential. When the time is right it is literally vital that such defences are challenged, unleashing potency, hope and a resparking of emotions, minds, and bodies. This is where we need to read another's nervous system and whisper to it and have the courage to help push through defences. Doing so can be vitalising, helping to grow zest for life, activating our lifegiver. Of course, all defences have been erected for good reasons, they require respect and will not to be let go off without a struggle; but we also need to know when to push through them.

In Khenan's case, his defence made sense as he had been bullied, abused, demeaned and in effect lost his mother when his stepfather came on the scene. He felt unlovable and had lost trust in adults. Like most children, he blamed himself when he was told off or rejected, feeling he was at fault, not the adults. He also knew to his cost how it could be dangerous to challenge or confront adults who were abusive such as his stepfather. Keeping a low profile, staying below the parapet, had served him well, but at a cost.

In one meeting he was talking about his stepfather and his breath quickened and legs started to move. I asked him what the feeling was towards his stepfather, was it anger? I asked if he could exaggerate the gesture and what he wanted to express. His immediate response was the classic 'learned helplessness' one, that it is best to keep his head down, not make a fuss. Khenan found it hard to believe that I could allow and hear his anger and help him express it. It was a bit easier with less serious incidents at school, such as being slighted or teased by another kid. Initially he would fudge his feelings, perhaps saying that what happened was 'unfair', but when pushed we could get nearer to real feelings like anger, even fury.

As we saw with Rana, he became more assertive. He was developing newfound confidence and becoming hopeful about possible changes. He began to stand up for himself in the playground, 'holding his ground', not taking things 'lying down', and as a result he felt more solid, with less need to elusively glide around. Such a shift can have more complicated repercussions for black youth. An action viewed as courageously assertive in a white middle class boy can be (mis)construed as threatening or dangerous in a young black man of the same age. It took courage from him, and support from me, to keep on growing in this way but the relief was palpable. He had a life now and a future. He even was no longer cowed by his stepfather, helped by how he was now bigger than him and had started seriously working out and learning boxing!

In cases like this bravery is required, in all parties. He needed to be challenged about his defensive manoeuvres, such as his compliant smile and evasive body gestures. It was hard for him to open up his chest, to stand up and be counted, express the rage, and upset bottled up inside him. Yet that is what frees up energy, give rise to sparking and makes one feel alive. In Khenan we saw an opening up, not closing down to life, a new litheness and muscularity, and once danger signals had given way to safeness, he developed a more capacious capacity to feel feelings he had previously pushed down. His priors were challenged, such as that things will always work out badly for him, that he would always lose in a fight, that no-one would like him, let alone find him attractive. With such changes, with feeling feelings he had previously not been able to know and own, I saw his psychosomatic symptoms like nausea, tics, and back problems recede considerably.

Summary

In this paper I have discussed why we need adaptations to our traditional technique when working with trauma, I have primarily focused on two distinct issues.

Firstly, I have suggested that after serious trauma, people often move into dissociated states, and when they are in such states they cannot begin to do the work of processing trauma until they know, at both a bodily and psychological level, that they can feel safe. Without this any attempt to process traumatic experiences can risk precipitating a re-traumatisation including PTSD symptoms such as flashbacks and bodily numbing. Once a sense of embodied safeness has been developed, then slowly more difficult experiences can begin to be processed. I suggest that in addition to the traditional psychoanalytic armamentarium, clinicians need to develop more capacity to understand and work at such a somatic level.

The second area where we might be challenged is in helping people express feelings which might be outside the usual psychoanalytic lexicon. In learned helplessness and some forms of depression, the lack of spark and vitality is due to a given-upness, a loss of hope and a dispiriting absence of belief in one's own agency. Both Rana and Khenan, arrived with a hopelessness deep in their beings. Through their therapy they both came back into their bodies, became outward facing, moving towards rather than away from life, developing the capacity to embrace a wider range of emotions.

Anger can be feared but is a vital force. The word aggression comes from the Latin, meaning to 'move towards', and in living a full life we can move towards experiences rather than away. That is a hallmark of resilience, as seen in brain science too (Davidson, 2000).

Anger and aggression are not an endpoint, but rather are often staging posts, often necessary ones, on the way to deeper feelings. Rana spent many hours in tears, experiencing grief about her early life, the loss of what was stolen, working through deep pain, as well as remorse for her poor relationship with her mother. These 'softer' feelings are I think only healthy when expressed in the right time and order. We can push the need to face depressive anxieties, sadness, grief, and pain too quickly, in a kind of short-cut, a therapeutic bypass, which avoids experiencing the rage and power that often needs to be felt first.

In both working with dissociative states, and in facilitating 'striated' muscle energetic power, I have found it necessary to be able to use much more awareness of somatic states than is usually developed in our formal trainings. I believe this to be an interesting challenge to take up in training therapists and in supervision.

Acknowledgements

I am grateful for being invited to give a Centenary lecture at the Tavistock Centre by and alongside my colleague Dr. Jo Stubley, where some of this material was highlighted.

Disclosure statement

No potential conflict of interest was reported by the author(s).

References

Abbass, A. (2015). *Reaching through resistance: Advanced psychotherapy techniques*. Seven Leaves Press.

Cuddy, A. (2015). *Presence: Bringing your boldest self to your biggest challenges*. Hachette.

Davanloo, H. (1979). Techniques of short-term dynamic psychotherapy. *Psychiatric Clinics of North America*, *2*(1), 11–22. https://doi.org/10.1016/S0193-953X(18)31021-9

Davidson, R. J. (2000). Affective style, psychopathology, and resilience: Brain mechanisms and plasticity. *The American Psychologist*, *55*(11), 1196–1214. https://doi.org/10.1037/0003-066X.55.11.1196

Fairbairn, W. R. D. (1962). *An object-relations theory of the personality*. Basic Books.

Ferenczi, S. (1926). *Final contributions to the problems and methods of psycho-analysis*. Karnac Books.

Fragkaki, I., Roelofs, K., Stins, J., Jongedijk, R. A., & Hagenaars, M. A. (2017). Reduced freezing in posttraumatic stress disorder patients while watching affective pictures. *Frontiers in Psychiatry*, *8*, 39. https://doi.org/10.3389/fpsyt.2017.00039

Garland, C. (2018). *Understanding trauma: A psychoanalytical approach* (pp. 9–31). Routledge.

Gilbert, P. (2019). Explorations into the nature and function of compassion. *Current Opinion in Psychology, 28*, 108–114. https://doi.org/10.1016/j.copsyc.2018.12.002

Kenrick, J., Lindsey, C., & Tollemache, L. (2006). *Creating new families: Therapeutic approaches to fostering, adoption, and kinship care*. Karnac Books.

Laing, R. D. (1969). *The divided self.* Pantheon Books New York.

Lanyado, M. (2003). *The presence of the therapist: Treating childhood trauma.* Routledge.

Maier, S. F., & Seligman, M. E. (1976). Learned helplessness: Theory and evidence. *Journal of Experimental Psychology: General, 105*(1), 3–46. https://doi.org/10.1037/0096-3445.105.1.3

Malan, D. H. (1976). *The frontier of brief psychotherapy: An example of the convergence of research and clinical practice.* Plenum Medical Book Co.

Music, G. (2019). *Nurturing children: Fro tramuma to growth using attachment theory, psychoanalysis and neurobiology.* Routledge.

Naviaux, R. K. (2020). Perspective: Cell danger response biology—the new science that connects environmental health with mitochondria and the rising tide of chronic illness. *Mitochondrion, 51*, 40–45. https://doi.org/10.1016/j.mito.2019.12.005

Ogden, P. (2006). *Trauma and the body: A sensorimotor approach to psychotherapy.* W. W. Norton & Co.

Parnell, L. (2013). *Attachment-focused EMDR: Healing relational trauma*. W. W. Norton & Company.

Reich, W. (1945). *Character analysis*. Straus and Giroux.

Van der Kolk, B. A. (2017). Developmental trauma disorder: Toward a rational diagnosis for children with complex trauma histories. *Psychiatric Annals, 35*(5), 401–408. https://doi.org/10.3928/00485713-20050501-06

Winnicott, D. W. (1971). *The use of an object and relating through identifications in playing and reality New York.* Basic Books.

Trauma and abuse

Judith Trowell

In this paper I reflect on my work with adult patients and the Tavistock based sexually abused girls study. I discuss two young women who came for help with their relationships, but subsequently disclosed having been sexually abused as children. I was particularly interested since contrary to what one might expect, the young woman who seemed to enjoy better relationship with her mother did less well in treatment. These two patients are contrasting and this underlines the importance of focussing on specific aspects of the primary maternal object relationship that are unique to each individual in understanding the ability to benefit from therapy. Important features shared across the two patients such as PTSD, the distortion of time, and the role of the father are considered. The timing of the disclosure is also an issue. Both patients elicit strong countertransference responses that were difficult to manage and the value of supervision was stressed. The author tries to address two questions, why the patient who had a better maternal relationship did not benefit as much, secondly the point in treatment when the disclosure occurred.

Introduction

As I look back over my clinical work in the field of abuse and trauma, I was reminded of the findings of the sexually abused girls study based at the Tavistock, and thinking about its helpfulness in my work with adult patients. I am left with two main questions that remained unanswered: first, how or why did the memory of being abused become accessible at a particular time; and, second, how might one understand the factors that led some patients to respond well to psychoanalytic treatment, while others did not? It is hoped this paper will be helpful to those working with similar patients.

Many authors have examined the effect of abuse on the structure and experience of time. Stubley (2013), in 'The Kraken Awakens', links trauma with particularities in the experience of time: 'how time is experienced is closely linked with understanding the nature of the trauma, loss of memory, phantasm and reality. Experiences are placed in a container. The container breaks open and floods out traumatic experiences' (p. 114). Perelberg (2007a) describes the complexity of Freud's notion of time, which includes developmental fixation, regression, repression, the return of the repressed, the timelessness of the unconscious, and *après coup* as axes of temporality. It does seem that understanding time, and how the mind – both conscious and unconscious – processes it, is significant, particularly where there has been trauma. Post-traumatic stress disorder (PTSD) involves flashbacks and re-experiencing, when the individual thinks the trauma is happening again. The unconscious functions differently from the conscious mind, splitting off the experience, which is either projected, leading to paranoia and aggression, or introjected and repressed, lost to consciousness and also to the possibility of emerging from the unconscious in an ordinary way. It is as though it had sunk into the 'deep' unconscious. This is beneath the usual sense of timelessness in the unconscious: it seems the experiences, sensations and memories become encapsulated and sink, like a stone in a bubble. The individual is left with depleted emotionality and gives an impression of flatness.

It should be noted the Royal Commission into Institutional Responses to Child Sexual Abuse in Australia (RCIRCSA, 2017) found that 42.6% of children disclosed in childhood, but if not then it could take 23.9 years before disclosure (females 20.5 years, males 25.7 years).

As well as PTSD, more subtle cognitive issues may be observed in connection with sexual abuse (and other kinds of trauma). Patients report that they cannot always focus their thoughts and that they move or jump from one idea or topic to the next. They realise that they have difficulty in maintaining a train of thought, which leaves them feeling that their minds run on or break up ideas. Symbolic capacity may be lost (Garland, 2004) so that concrete thinking is all that remains. Symbolic capacity is key to being able to consider issues from different perspectives, to play with ideas and thoughts, or to learn. With the loss of it, the patient is left thinking in two dimensions, in a flat, concrete way.

Following trauma, some losses are inevitable – for example, the loss of loved ones, of one's home, of the capacity to work. Most powerfully, there is the loss of innocence and trust, of the underlying sense that the world is basically a good place (Lemma & Levy, 2004). They may struggle with the emotional flatness that comes with dissociation (Bronstein, 2020), as intense feelings that threaten to overwhelm them are split off and evacuated, or taken deeper inside the unconscious. These defensive processes leave patients depleted of feelings. There is loss of personal integrity and of the sense of self, which is a profound aspect of trauma and can lead to despair. Patients are left confused and struggling. However, it is important to acknowledge the courage and intelligence of many trauma survivors who nevertheless manage to try to make sense of what has happened and to get on with their lives.

I will discuss some of these considerations in relation to two patients.

In the first case, it emerged that the father was very present but was sadomasochistic as well as the reported perpetrator of actual sexual abuse. In the second case, the father was often absent; he could be violent, though the abuse she suffered was not carried out by him, but he could also be caring and concerned. These patients were left feeling that they were helpless and that they had to endure whatever happened. This can lead to hopelessness and, underlying this, to fury. Their lives had been damaged, and there is no way that they can go back and have a fresh start to an early life which does not leave them damaged and troubled.

But perhaps the most profound and most difficult experience, both for the patient and for the analyst, is the experience of intrapsychic loss: the damage to the internal world caused by the absence of an internal creative, caring parental couple. Frequently, particularly in the case of sexual abuse, there is a failure to resolve the oedipal conflict (given the inappropriate sexual contact), and it is this loss that, in recovery, becomes in many ways overwhelming. The work in this situation needs to focus on giving up the illusion of an exclusive relationship with the parent and then on relinquishing the internal abusive relationship.

The sexually abused girls study

The second question (concerning which cases do well in treatment) may, perhaps, be considered in the light of an outcome study on work with sexually abused girls (Trowell et al., 2002). This was part of a research project at the Tavistock Clinic that was set up to explore whether girls who had been sexually abused could benefit from psychoanalytic psychotherapy. The material referred to arose from this study involving the Tavistock Clinic, the Maudsley Children's Dpartment, Camberwell Child Guidance Clinic, the Royal Free Hospital and Great Ormond Street hospital.

The project offered up to 30 sessions of individual psychotherapy with parent work or psycho educational group therapy to girls between 6 years and 14 years. The patients were randomly allocated to each of the therapeutic interventions. All of the parents or carers of the girls were offered support and parent work (Rushton & Miles, 2000). All the individual therapists received regular supervision in pairs and the two group therapists were also supervised, two for each group. The therapists were asked to keep detailed process notes, and sessions were audio taped.

When detailed process notes of the once-weekly sessions with the girls were submitted to qualitative analysis (Long & Trowell, 2001), it was found that the girls who did well according to standardized outcome measures were those whose parents engaged with the treatment process, and also where the therapists had addressed the negative transference in connection with termination. It needs to be emphasized that these girls received once-weekly therapy for 30 sessions only, whereas both the adult patients I discuss here were seen three times weekly (and sometimes four times weekly) on an ongoing basis. In other words, any extrapolation from the children to the adult patients must be subject to a consideration of several important differences: of frequency and length of treatment and of age, as well as the resulting fact that the girls' parents still exerted an important direct influence on them and on the treatment process, whereas with the adults this influence was exerted by the patients' internal parental figures.

Analysis of the notes from the girls' therapy suggested that there were three groups within this sample. Those in the first group could retrieve a protective and available object during the psychotherapy. This group were living in settled families, where the abuser was from the extended family or was a close family friend, and the abuse was taken seriously (Brenman, 2006). Those in the second group showed only a limited capacity to retrieve an emotionally available object or to experience one in therapy. These girls came from dysfunctional families, where the abuse was ignored or was an additional problem. In this group there was more intrafamilial abuse by fathers, brothers or cousins. The third group were in chaotic situations with no obvious parental care, and they revealed a continuing experience of fragmented or bizarre objects. Those girls who failed to improve with the psychotherapy on offer were all in this third group.

Implications for clinical work

These research findings, as I have noted, cannot be directly translated to a conceptualization of my adult patients in intensive treatment, but they have helped me to think about the presentations with which I have been confronted. I think that, in the midst of the experience of powerful degrees of mindlessness, projective identification and intense feeling, they have allowed me to hold on to both my psychoanalytic understanding and my awareness of the impact of trauma: this is particularly difficult to manage where the body boundary has actually been breached, as is the case in sexual abuse. This involvement of the body leads to a complex psychological response: a particular form of emotional abuse, perhaps because of the perversion alongside the lies and threats that accompany it (Trowell, 1988).

In all our work supervision is essential but never more so than in these case when abuse emerges, one may need additional consultations to understand and manage the work.

The two adult patients I consider provide an opportunity to explore the possible long-term consequences of abuse in early life. The impact of such experiences is indeed generally thought to be long-lasting. It is also my aim to consider the two patients' capacity to make good use of psychoanalytic work and, in this way, to approach my second question.

The first patient I discuss grew up in a family where some good-enough early parenting was present. This, however, later became corrupted by the influence of a sadomasochistic parental relationship, which, in the patient's account, was dominated by paranoia, triumph, cruelty and hatred. The father was described as exerting tyrannical control over his family; the mother seemed to accept this, or perhaps even went along with the perverse activity.

The second patient had had very little early parenting, surviving by finding fragments of care from those around her (neighbours, an aunt and a shadowy father). Her internal world consisted of bits and pieces, bizarre objects – mainly part-objects and perhaps an early vague whole-object, which may have been what gave her the hope to seek treatment. Apparently, her mother had serious mental health problems and was said to spend most of her time in bed. The first patient, then, could superficially seem to resemble the second group of girls – those who had a limited capacity to access a good internal figure during therapy – whereas the second patient more nearly resembled the girls in the chaotic third group. However, a closer look at the two adult patients' material shows that these external resemblances do not go far enough in accounting for their different outcomes in treatment, and that it is necessary to consider this in the light of the more subtle features of their relationship to their primary internal figures, as revealed in the transference relationship. Significantly, these features also have an important bearing on my first question: that is, on the timing of their disclosure of abuse.

During my assessment I regularly ask if anything unpleasant or frightening has ever happened. If yes I ask for more details and ask about touching,holding, hitting and encourage the individual to say more, they often worry you do not want to hear. In these cases nothing emerged at this stage.

I consult to a network of local schools from whence came the referrals.

The first patient, 'Sonia', had had some good early experiences but many adverse ones, so that emotional deprivation was a factor in this case. At the age of 29, she said that she was worried she could not sustain relationships. She worked as a junior-school teacher and was restless at work; she felt she was not doing a sufficiently good job. Her early life had been difficult. She was the younger of two daughters, and she felt her parents had wanted a boy. Her parents did not get on: there had been lots of disagreements and domestic violence, and she and her sister were sometimes caught in the crossfire. I felt that she was an intelligent woman, but there was something strange about her. She had no mental health history, but mother and maternal grandmother had been depressed. I felt concerned for her vulnerability, but I did not feel involved: there was no warmth between us. I felt that I was being distanced – or was I distancing myself? We arranged that she would come three times weekly on the way to school, but this soon increased to four times a week, because she found the breaks difficult to manage. She had had early good-enough mothering: her mother had loved her as a baby but withdrew when she started school. Her maternal grandfather was a benign frequent presence and fulfilled a good paternal role. This suggested that the lack of proper alignment of the generations may have contributed to the distortion of her sense of time. The intergenerational confusion inevitably involved this patient in losing an appropriate understanding in her internal world of the time boundaries of the generations.

A Thursday session, after six months
Sonia started at once:

P: 'It has been a tough week. As a child the feelings were so powerful and yet no one ever confirmed that the sneering, the mocking, the contempt, the way what was said leapt out at you, got right inside you. Nothing was ever said.'
T: 'I wonder if you are saying that you are unsure what is internal and what external.'
P: 'Yes, if there is a crisis at work then I am OK, but here it slips. I lose any sense of myself, things get right inside me.'

I had a strong reaction to her previous statement, and her acknowledgement that her capacity to keep thoughts and feelings at bay here made me wonder what she was struggling to avoid. She seemed to fear that in the transference there was an opening up of her mind to memories as yet undisclosed.

T: 'I am wondering now when you say, "got right inside you", if something really did?'

I said this because for some weeks I had been increasingly uncomfortable: there was something not spoken, withheld; and in that moment it felt there on the surface.

P: 'When he was in those moods, he had me go to the bedroom, and yes, he did put his thing inside me. But what I cannot understand is why she never did anything, why she went on taking his rage, and letting him take me. Why did she not stand up to him? She never stood her ground, never told him to shut up, or refuse to do whatever he wanted. I realised he was sort of mental, sick.'
T: 'It sounds as though you had to face that she was, in a way, in it, too.'
P: 'Yes, she could have answered back. It was so awful, she could have left, gone to stay with her parents, taken us with her, if she could not fight.

We were able to think about the sadomasochism of the parents and how it was repeated in our transference relationship and in the here and now. She could see how she had dismissed me as being of little help and had at times been critical and mocked me. She also had to face her recognition of her father's penetrative abuse of her. It felt at that point as though we were in touch, as though I could be there for her.

T: 'Up until now you have seen your mother as the vulnerable, abused mother, and you tried to protect her, but now you are talking about someone who went along with it, did not prevent his abuse of you.'
P: 'Yes, and she is still doing it. The façade was so different, a nice, together family walking through the village to church on Sundays. That was his weapon. If I ever tried to say anything, he would say "well, Jesus says honour your father and mother", endless bloody sermons.'

The following weeks and months were grim. There were sessions where she was beside herself, believing her father knew she had told me about the abuse and that he was outside peering in. The abuser was now felt to be outside – presumably to protect the analyst from being experienced as the abuser. She often saw his face in the window and expected him to be waiting outside when she left. Sometimes she stayed silent throughout. She came from the north of England, so there was little likelihood in reality of him being outside. Traumatised patients have flashbacks, and it is not easy to distinguish a flashback from a hallucination. With this patient, the face of her father was a hallucination, but a pseudo-hallucination, because she was aware that the image came from within her own mind; it was not actually there, although at times it felt briefly real, a transient psychotic moment. Trying to understand this, it is possible to think that allowing herself to tell me about events with her parents opened up split-off experiences; she then needed to protect them from her rage.

At times I felt puzzled, as though she did know he was not really there, but at other times it was so real and vivid that I, too, looked at the window for his face and wondered if he was there, however unlikely I knew it to be. The transient psychotic moment held me too, and I resonated to her terror.

She had missed a session and was insisting there was little I could offer to her that was helpful. The capacity to deny herself, the double deprivation (Williams, 1997) was obvious, but also the attack on me: the atmosphere felt sadomasochistic. It was not only her denial that I might have something helpful to offer, it was the relentless disparagement, the dismissal of whatever I said, that left me feeling useless. My feelings were of hopelessness and anger: her contempt was so powerful that I felt perhaps she was right, and someone else might do better. With hindsight, I would understand this as reflecting at least in part her own feelings of worthlessness, both in relation to her parents in general and to the abuse in particular.

A session some months later

At this point, the patient was wanting to plan finishing treatment.

She arrived about 4 minutes late, came in quite rapidly and eagerly lay down. There was a feeling of agitation.

P: 'I was thinking, driving here, how awful it will be when I do not have here anymore, how will I keep myself together, and yet I am also reluctant to keep on coming, it is hard to make myself get up so early.'

T: 'So partly a relief to allow yourself to think that one day you will not have this very early start, but also you feel very anxious and frightened. But I am struck that it seems to be feeling quite imminent, and I am wondering about that, because as I understand it we are continuing.'

P: 'Yes, we are, but I think it is even thinking that it will end one day.'

This seems to indicate that when there is something stressful, then her sense of time evaporates, as though her father is coming between us to control her.

She demonstrates that as soon as she thinks something, it is felt to be happening. This is a coalescence of impulse and event, which disguises her own wishes and feelings. It came about by her longing to be close and special to father, but then came anxiety and agitation when her own ordinary oedipal wish seemed to be confirmed by the abuse, apparently erasing the distinction between her internal world and outside reality, the thought that she came between her parents, and that her father favoured her. She could not allow herself to think about the intimate relationship between her parents.

> P: 'My thinking so easily fragments, I cannot connect anything, cannot think straight, I become confused and muddled. I could so easily revert to that, the way I used to be. The danger is I will just withdraw.'

It is worth recognising how the patient's thoughts about our ending became condensed. The time between our discussion and the ending actually happening disappeared, so that it felt imminent.

> T: 'In order to avoid the sadness and the pain, I suppose I am wondering about this avoiding sadness.'
> P: 'I am usually just glad to go and never give it a thought, I never expect anyone to remember me, that I did anything good.'

This recurrent plea for reassurance and to know that she mattered was an invitation to join the sadomasochistic dance unless I was careful. She could triumph if I sought to insist that, of course, I remember her, think about her.

> T: 'So talk of sadness may really be a fear of being forgotten, that I will be glad to see you go.'

We set a date to finish a year later, and she ended treatment as planned. She had a more senior post and had been with her current partner for more than two years. But her ending did feel rather like a cutting off: there was no sadness, no real goodbye: she just went. I was left sad and concerned for her; my comment that I would be here if she needed me was ignored.

She had arrived in a frozen state, withdrawn, suspicious and terribly unhappy, but it was I who was left finding the sadness of separation hard to bear. I felt concern for her – there was so much more work to do – but I also felt a failure, that I had no value, had nothing to offer her. The sexual abuse, when it emerged, was not talked about in detail, but had a powerful emotional impact. In the transference I was the powerful, cruel father, or the mother who turned a blind eye to her distress and suffering. Like her father, I became an analyst who was triumphing over her, and it was hard to modify; it was her fantasy, and it was difficult to address, contain and thereby reduce its intensity. Her loss of the thoughtful, caring analyst opened up the fact of the loss of her family, her home, her capacity to trust; perhaps it was that she had never before had the loss of a relationship where trust had been present, to whatever degree. Loss of the analyst as a good object opened up her earlier deprivations. It was very hard for her to be able to bear her thoughts; for her to face her mindlessness, her terror and a sense of something repulsive about what she had gone through, or of herself as repulsive. (In reality, I felt defeated by her rather than repulsed.) The terror of her father, and the pseudo-hallucinations, were hard to contain alongside times when the sense of evil was projected into me: I became the cruel abuser delighting in her terror. She was often silent, but she did keep coming. Very slowly, we could work together on all this.

Slowly the splitting and projective identification lessened, and she could acknowledge her fear of me and her rage with me. I became less the cruel analyst/father or the mother who refused to see her distress. I think throughout we both knew that although her mind 'played tricks on her', she could hold on to reality outside the consulting room. There was something about coming too close to the experience in the transference that made her lose her sense of distance or symbolic capacity. She owned her own sexuality and enjoyed being a woman for the first time, but I did not feel we were able to bring together and fully release her potential and her creativity.

Sonia terminated her therapy with many unresolved issues. The losses she could mourn, and she could recognise the deprivation, but her rage and murderousness, although modified, remained. She would have needed to allow herself to really engage and commit to her therapy, but perhaps it was too hard while needing to work and function. She might have needed to be in a place that could care for her for a while. I felt she had gone as far as she could at that time, but that her underlying personality difficulties felt unresolved and would need further work. I learnt some years later that she had serious mental health difficulties.

The research with the sexually abused girls helped me to think about Sonia, an adult who had been abused in childhood. At the start, before her disclosure, she could have been in the first of the three groups; when we knew of the dysfunctional family, she fell into the second group. The abuse, when it came to the surface, showed how this patient had had some good maternal care early in her life and had an internal world with internal objects, however perverse.

Thinking about the questions which I pose in this paper, the timing of the abuse surfacing was about six months in to her analysis. She had begun to see me as a potentially good object. This seems consistent with reports in the literature that indicate individuals need to build up trust before they can share these experiences. The second question was whether she could really use her work with me. This felt only partly possible: her fear of a full psychotic breakdown may have prevented her or perhaps the psychic fractures would have been beyond outpatient help.

Second patient

The second patient, 'Mary', might have fallen into the third category of girls in the research project, from a chaotic situation, she, unlike Sonia, had never really had any psychological or emotional parenting: even food, clothing and accommodation had been poor. This left an internal world that consisted of fragments, although her intellectual capacity meant that she had managed to become an outwardly functioning person. Seriously troubled, this patient had had very little parental care, learning to manage herself and her (younger) sibling. She immediately made an intense, positive, idealising transference to me, which moved very rapidly into becoming demanding and controlling when I had breaks or had to change sessions. Her response to breaks, absences and frustrations could be extreme; but her complaint was that she did not get enough from me, rather than that I was useless or was abusing her. She was able to complain that I was an insufficiently present mother, rather than one who failed to protect her against an abusive father.

Mary came to treatment in her late thirties. She was divorced with no children, and, like Sonia, she worked as a primary school teacher. She was very keen to have help and had some insight. She was the elder of two children and had been taken into care at the age of nearly 5 years, when her mother and father separated and disappeared: neither would take the children. They were placed with different families, and she was quite seriously neglected, both physically and emotionally. Her development was delayed. She had had little toilet training and was used to looking for food for herself and her younger sibling.

Her relationship with her birth mother, such as it was, had consisted of mother making demands on her to sort out the little one. Mother was in bed a lot: Mary as an adult saw her as having mental and physical health problems. Father was violent to his wife and the children, but he did also provide some care. This was supplemented by an aunt and neighbours. Mary did not have an internal world with whole objects: the mother seemed to be all bad, father was both good and bad, caring but violent when there, but often absent. But she did seem to have had a (pre?)conception of a good object that was not there, and she reproached me for not being there sufficiently rather than denigrating me.

Foster carers had found Mary hard to manage, and she was moved several times. In her second placement, the elder birth son in the family abused her sexually for some 24 months. She mentioned it to a friend at school, who told her mother, and when the mother reported it, she was moved again. The final foster placement lasted. They could tolerate her behaviour, and she was there from the age of 9. As an adult, she remained in touch with them: she visited them, and they came to her wedding. She developed academically and became attached to her foster carers and their family, but she remained troubled by any intimacy and had issues with her gender identity: in many ways she saw herself as a boy. She had no sense of a maternal figure.

Nor was there a sense of a creative couple in her mind. She seemed identified with a father who had taken an interest in her, who attended school functions when he could, and whom she had continued to see as an adult, whereas her mother had disappeared. Being female was linked in her mind to shit, her younger sibling's and her mother's: she had had to clean them all up. The shit part of herself was projected onto me or appeared in her dreams. The feminine part of herself was rejected unconsciously; the masculine part was more evident and was an acknowledged part of her. In adolescence she enjoyed going around in a group, but when couples began pairing off, she found it hard. She was an attractive young woman, and the boys fancied her, so she went down the route of boyfriends, eventually marrying one of them at the age of 25. However, as the novelty wore off and the pressure to have children grew, she became increasingly distressed. She could not cope with the demands and expectation of her femaleness, which to her meant having babies and a family life and giving up her work and independence. It seemed to me that, even more than this, she feared the intimacy of family life. Finally, she and her husband divorced, and she had been on her own for about three years when she came for treatment.

The early sessions were full of the divorce and attempts to find her sibling and to trace her mother. Father had died. The loss of her mother was very painful: how could she have left? Why did she never make contact? Mary tried to understand, but her longing and fury were palpable. She had started in once-weekly therapy and then went up to twice weekly. For a short period she came four times a week, which is when the abuse emerged.

A session after two and a half years of treatment

This session was on a Monday just before my two-week Easter break it illustrates her neediness and desperation.

P: 'I don't know where to start, I hate the last week before the break. Can you help?'
T: 'I suppose I am wondering why it is so hard today in particular.'
P: 'Because I'm thinking all the time that you will not be here next week.'
T: 'So it feels there is no point starting today.'
P: 'NO, it is just that I cannot bear it, I cannot bear it, and these years of therapy make no difference, all this holding in mind, remembering, going on being, coming back. Nothing makes any difference, and you just do not understand. I CAN'T BEAR IT. Why don't you make it bearable by not expecting me to be able to manage? I cannot cope with breaks – what do I have to do to make you understand, commit suicide? I cannot cope.'
T: 'You feel totally overwhelmed, abandoned by me, dropped.'
P: 'Yes, but the words make no difference, I know it is like my mother leaving, and you are not her, but I just feel it every time.'

(Again, as with Sonia, the symbolic aspect of the transference felt unsustainable at crisis points.)

T: 'So my understanding the terror, the fear, the desperation, the panic and that we can talk about it does not help?'
P: 'No, it doesn't.'

The loss and deprivation here are unthinkable. It is an act of cruelty on my part, my ruthless indifference, but it is also her omnipotent belief that I can be controlled. My guilt and my rage at feeling trapped were difficult to manage, I wanted and needed to escape.

After the break, which she survived, she fairly quickly told me that she remembered the sexual abuse. This was new to me: she had not mentioned it during the assessment or previous sessions. It is as though she conflated the 'abuse' of my break with being penetrated or displaced by a phallic element that she may have felt was linked to me during my absence. If so, this resembles Sonia's situation in that the abuse came up at the point that a masculine element appeared in her transference experience of me. In Mary's case, the 'bad' masculine part seemed to separate her from a 'good' me, whereas for Sonia I became this bad part.

At this point, I was useless, as I was for Sonia, but I had a different response, which indicates what she is reproaching me for. My reaction with Mary was to feel sucked dry, as though I could never offer enough. My dread, revulsion, and outrage as she attempted to control me were very hard to contain. Perhaps my different countertransference in each case provided a clue to my patients' respective central problem of good object absent as opposed to bad object present (O'Shaughnessy, 2015).

A session a few weeks later illustrates Mary's intense neediness and her desperate attempts to control me.

She started immediately:

P: 'I dreamt I had to go to the doctor for a smear, she told me to get undressed and put my legs up. I did this, and she came over, everything was ok. I thought, I have got this far and it seems OK, I thought I could talk to her. I thought I could tell her she could not do the smear because there was something wrong with me. She said it would be OK, and I was not to worry.
I said she didn't understand, she did not realise that there really was something wrong with me, something wrong with my vagina.
I said to the doctor, if she went ahead she would tear me apart, could she just find out what was wrong with me. She said there is no problem, she put the speculum inside and said, look, it is fine. I started screaming at her that she did not understand, that there was something wrong, and if she opened the speculum it would tear me apart. I screamed.

This was a desperate, primitive feeling – perhaps that separation between sessions felt like being torn apart bodily in a way that links to sexual abuse or rape. Her rage and hatred and yet her passionate longing to be understood left her desperately needy.

After she reported the dream, there was a silence.

P: 'Why don't you speak?'
T: 'I was thinking about the dream and wondering what your thoughts were.'
P: 'Well, I thought about when I was young with that second foster family. I kept saying this is not alright. He didn't listen; in the end I told my teacher, and then I was moved and it stopped.
T: 'You stopped it, so there is something about this woman doctor/analyst: Will she listen, does she understand, or will she, without realising, tear you apart?'
Silence.
P: 'Can you talk please.'

The barrage of emotional demands and the distress and resentment it produced in me went on for over a year. My concern and compassion were taken to the limit. Without supervision, I could not have continued. The dread of each session and what I had to cope with and survive, and my revulsion at some of the sexual material, were very powerful. How to gradually untangle the agony of the loss of her birth family and times in care and the impact of the sexual abuse in one of the placements? Perhaps they had such a powerful effect because they weren't distinguished: they coalesced for her, as the abuse is how she experienced the absence. The mourning and the longing to go back and have a different childhood were desperately present in the room.

Another issue was myself as a woman. At times she felt it would be easier to talk to a man: why had she come to a woman, then a woman psychiatrist who was driving her mad? I struggled with her rage, hatred and passionate longing. It was hard to have a life of my own, she often filled my head, and dislodging her was almost impossible. Her capacity to work on the material and to face it did make me admire her courage and determination. But her fear was ever-present: fear that she could not bear the rage and hate that swept over her, and over myself at times. I am aware that my countertransference was very powerful and that my own emotions and response were very apparent to her.

The timing of her disclosure of the abuse was later, after a break 36 months into her analysis, but in this case it seemed it was a fragment of her trauma, the loss of her home, her family, her mother, that was the overwhelming issue for her. In both cases, where I was in the transference makes sense of the timing of the disclosure. Gradually she became able to use what was on offer, but the toll on me was extreme. But her bravery and intelligence carried one along.

Discussion

Perhaps the most profound problem for these traumatised patients, and the most difficult for patient and analyst, was the experience of loss: the intrapsychic loss and damage to their internal worlds. In sexual abuse there is a failure of any resolution of the oedipal conflict, and it is this loss that, during recovery, can become overwhelming. Britton (2013) states that 'the work needs to focus on the identification and then relinquishment of the relationship with each parent so there is the emergence of a triangular space. This then allows the patient to individuate and separate' (p. 86).

In these cases time is one of the central issues that needs to be managed. When the body boundary has actually been infringed, does it distort the capacity to place things in time? Papers in *Time and Memory* (Perelberg, 2007b) indicate that it does. There can be distortion of sequencing, or condensation where there is blurring of events into one occasion. Certainly, very intense feelings are projected, but the struggle to hold on to what was then, what is now and what might be is particularly difficult. In the unconscious, timelessness holds sway: events may not be sequenced, so that distortion occurs easily. Repression, projection, splitting and denial are the usual mechanisms used in abuse, but here we can see excessive use, leaving the individuals with very limited resources to cope with life. Regression easily occurs, as seen in the second case, Mary, with dependence and demands. The timing of the return of the repressed or split-off experiences is still unclear, making it uncertain when a disclosure will occur.

Disclosure of sexual abuse is mostly rather tentative in on going work. As the clinician, one may have had various comments that could be clues. More often one has a sinking feelings thought that something nasty is being projected. Then there is a moment when it comes together and one can say, put into words, the thought of inappropriate sexual activity. In these two cases the first was such a case, in the second it felt the holiday break cracked open a memory that surfaced on her return.

Both my patients had lost a sense of themselves as individuals. They struggled with terror and anxiety – the anxiety of going on being (Winnicott, 1956, p. 303), or anxieties-of-being (Durban, 2017). This was a deep layer of anxiety, because there was something profoundly absent, particularly for Mary, but also for Sonia. As Durban (2017, p. 186) states,

> the destruction of the external home ... reflects the loss of contact with an internal supportive relationship. This loss severely damages the capacity to tolerate and endure psychic pain, leading to an inability to mourn and to a stubborn avoidance of knowing, resulting in mindlessness.

Neither patient felt that they had a home or a family: they felt rootless, and the longing and the neediness were very painful. Sonia coped by cutting off, and I felt distanced. Mary, in contrast, wanted to become part of my family, and the envy and rage when exclusion confronted her at the end of sessions and in the breaks were very hard to bear. The sense of absence was overwhelming, and the weekends, the holiday breaks, the gaps between sessions, all became engulfed in a sense of being lost in space and ceasing to exist. It felt like an experience of time being frozen, so that the torment would go on forever.

Finding a way to help both patients to face their losses, to begin to mourn that which was and that which could never be, to begin to move from concrete thinking to symbolic functioning, was a slow, painful struggle, with limited success. The impact on me was considerable. With Sonia, I was constantly being tested: could I bear her contempt and fury, and the communication of her feeling unlikeable? In the countertransference, she felt distant from herself and me, and yet she was acutely aware of any moment when my attention slipped. I felt battered and abused, penetrated by her rage, as well as, sometimes, outraged at being treated like that; and I had to struggle with managing what I came to recognise as the sadistic father who was lodged in me. Momentary glimpses of her vulnerability and neediness seemed very obvious, though she dismissed them immediately.

With Mary, on the other hand, her endless demands, her overwhelming need, and her determination to impose her will made it impossible at times to be clear about what was then, what was now, and what was the immediate future. It became impossible to think: the intensity of the projective identifications left me mindless and blown away, penetrated by her demands, as all the many past losses were focused on me in the here and now.

How might one understand the different outcomes achieved by these two patients?

Both Sonia and Mary came to treatment with 'ordinary' problems; they had developed careers and aspired to relationships. But in fact, the deprivation and emotional abusive aspect of the sexual abuse had undermined their sense of personhood. In the countertransference my genuine concern was easily turned into dislike and hatred, and this was difficult to work through. This perversion of love was a reflection of the impossibility of trust.

Of the two patients, Mary was the more disturbed and damaged under her functioning exterior. The lack of basic parenting meant there had been little early containment. The intense emotional outpouring of hate, longing, loving, needing and greed filled me for months. But the slow and gradual processing that I eventually found possible (Brenman Pick, 1992) and our capacity to find spaces to work did enable her to take in a mind that could think and make sense of her experiences. Sonia was also functioning in the external world but was damaged and traumatised. Her early mothering had been to some extent protective, which suggested that she could have used her analysis. But this did not happen: she took refuge from her internalised sadistic father and weak, complicit mother by turning to a rigid psychic retreat or a pseudo-autistic state that proved impossible to penetrate. Sonia was not able to think about her need: she used an autistic straitjacket (Tustin, 1990) to protect herself.

Britton (2003, p. 70) states that 'for psychic balance we need two internal parents, whatever the case in the outside world' (p. 70). Marks (2002, p. 98) states: 'The capacity for symbol representation depends on the development of an ability to discriminate the other from the self and then represent mentally in its absence … usually the father' (p. 98). These two women's fathers were rather different. Sonia had a father, but not a loving, caring father: rather, a sadistic and abusive man; he used his family to enact his rage and destructiveness and used his power to dominate. With Mary, an inadequate father could not cope with his children, and they were placed in care. Mary responded to the interest and care from the older foster brother but then had to face the fact that her father substitute was not what he had seemed. Both women as girls had to face the realisation that the men in their lives did not see them as individuals but as objects for their own gratification; they projected into the girls their triumph and contempt. For Sonia, it seemed impossible to achieve any distance from the sadistic father lodged in her mind, so that she remained in a state of concrete equivalence with him, with no possibility of symbolisation. For Mary, on the other hand, the capacity to symbolise grew, and a violent but more vulnerable father in her mind slowly emerged.

These two patients shared a profound failure very early on in their development: symbolic capacity had not been developed at a deep internal level (Garland, 2002). Separation had not taken place psychically, and there was little actual containment provided. In Sonia there was some capacity to think, a space, so that some early experience had provided some containing capacity. For Mary, it seemed there was initially only concrete thinking and very little symbolic capacity, and she was primarily sensation-driven. Durban (2017, p. 186), states 'thinking about these early anxiety states ... these anxieties of being include the experiences of having no body, existing solely through the senses which are often mixed and dislocated, having no inside or outside, leaking out and emptying ... and having no sense of time or space'.

What was overwhelming in their behaviour was very different: Sonia projected uselessness/contempt, a bad internal object, Mary raged against me for my absence. In other words, she had an idea of good object absent, which Sonia did not, and this presumably links to her better outcome. So, too, may be the fact that it wasn't her father who had carried out the abuse, and she, unlike Sonia, had been believed.

How does this link to my introductory thoughts about the girls in the research project and to my two initial questions? Sonia, my first case, initially appeared to have had some good experiences, but this became more obviously fragmenting, and the lengthy destructive relationships in her family left her isolated and unreachable. Her decision to finish therapy after a few years left her still in her withdrawn state.

Both young women were seriously damaged. The first, stuck in her paranoid-schizoid state, wanted but could not leave her psychic retreat. The second, after a long and desperate struggle, had some future possibilities.

In the outcome study of the girls, it seemed to be the family structure that affected the different outcomes, but in these two adults the case was rather different. What saved Sonia's life was her ability to develop a cut-off state: in the countertransference she evacuated her sense of being useless that kept me as useless, unable to offer anything helpful. I was able perhaps to do some reasonable work around the edges, but her sense of triumph remained: her hatred could not be metabolised.

Mary's neediness was apparent in every way, and the countertransference was overwhelming at times. The projective identification evoked in me guilt that I could not provide what she needed but also awareness nothing would ever be enough. I felt overwhelmed and wanted to escape, but I also knew it was a growth-promoting process that we had to live through, and she did finally manage a stable, solid relationship (I think) with a male colleague.

What does this mean for analysts taking on such cases? Initially, Sonia seemed likely to be able to use analysis; however, her apparently intact family was so controlled by the parental sadomasochistic system dominant in her internal world that she could not break free. Perhaps, had she been an inpatient, it might have been possible, but as an outpatient she did not have the capacity to undertake such a fundamental and frightening path. Mary, on the other hand, while having so much ground to make up, was, perhaps, in some ways less damaged by the almost total neglect, with the trauma and abuse in addition. She was left able to use, over a length of time, the help on offer. In other words, the facts of the abusive incidents in themselves do not fully explain the outcome.

I hope this paper can contribute something to those struggling with these tragic cases and may provide a way of understanding the psychopathology of such patients and their capacity to use, or not, the help we can offer. It is also clear that for an adult abused when a child, the disclosure rarely comes initially. It is often after six months or more (RCIRCSA, 2017), perhaps after a break, a weekend or holiday break, that a disclosure may be triggered. In these two cases it was after 6 months and 36 months, respectively. What does this mean for analysts taking on patients? Perhaps it suggests that however careful we are with the initial assessment, we cannot predict what might emerge in the course of the work. We need to be prepared for an eruption of intense emotions that at times feels almost impossible to contain and threatens to sweep away analyst and patient.

I can only repeat how important it is to have supervision in place. It is important for all our cases, as it is hard to predict what may emerge during the course of the work and when the supervision can become a life-saver. It is also important to remember that following sexual abuse, we can help the psychic wound heal, but a scar is left.

Disclosure statement

No potential conflict of interest was reported by the author(s).

References

Brenman Pick, I. (1992). The emergence of early object relations in the psychoanalytic setting. In F. Davids & N. Shavit (Eds.), *Authenticity in the psychoanalytic encounter: The work of Irma Brenman Pick* (pp. 38–47). Routledge.

Brenman, E. (2006). *Recovery of the lost good object*. Routledge.

Britton, R. S. (2003). *Sex, death, and the superego*. Karnac.
Britton, R. S. (2013). External danger and threat. In E. McGinley & A. Varchevker (Eds.), *Enduring trauma through the life cycle* (pp. 90). Routledge.
Bronstein, C. (2020). Psychosis and psychotic functioning in adolescence. *The International Journal of Psychoanalysis*, *101*(1), 136–151. https://doi.org/10.1080/00207578.2020.1720146
Durban, J. (2017). Home, homelessness and nowhere-ness in early infancy. *Journal of Child Psychotherapy*, *43*(2), 175–191. https://doi.org/10.1080/0075417X.2017.1327550
Garland, C. (2002). *Understanding trauma*. Karnac.
Garland, C. (2004). Traumatic events and their impact on symbolic functioning. In S. Levy & A. Lemma (Eds.), *The perversion of loss: Psychoanalytic perspectives on trauma* (pp. 37–49). Whurr.
Lemma, A., and Levy, S. (2004). Introduction. In S. Levy & A. Lemma (Eds.), *The perversion of loss: Psychoanalytic perspectives on trauma* (pp. xv). Whurr.
Long, J., & Trowell, J. (2001). Individual brief psychotherapy with sexually abused girls. *Psychoanalytic Psychotherapy*, *15*(1), 39–59. https://doi.org/10.1080/02668730100700031
Marks, M. (2002). Letting fathers in. In J. Trowell & A. Etchegoyen (Eds.), *The importance of fathers: A psychoanalytic re-evaluation* (pp. 98). Routledge.
O'Shaughnessy, E. (2015). The absent object. In R. Rusbridger (Ed.), *Inquiries in psychoanalysis: Collected papers of Edna O'Shaughnessy* (pp. 19-31). Routledge.
Perelberg, R. (2007a). Introduction. In R. J. Perelberg (Ed.), *Time and memory* (pp. xiii-xxi). Karnac.
Perelberg, R. (2007b). Space and time in psychoanalytic listening. *The International Journal of Psychoanalysis*, *88*(6), 1473–1490. https://doi.org/10.1516/VG65-8L74-2317-8492
RCIRCSA. (2017). *Royal Commission into Institutional Responses to Child Sexual Abuse. Final report, Volume 4: Identifying and disclosing child sexual abuse*. Commonwealth of Australia
Rushton, A., & Miles, G. (2000). A study of support services for the current carers of sexually abused girls. *Clinical Child Psychology and Psychicry*, *5*(3), 411–426. https://doi.org/10.1177/1359104500005003010
Stubley, J. (2013). The Kraken awakens: The re-emergence of traumatic experiences when defences break down. In E. McGinley & A. Varchevker (Eds.), *Enduring trauma through the life cycle* (pp. 114). Karnac.
Trowell, J., Kolvin, I., Weeramanthri, T., Sadowski, H., Berelowitz, M., Glaser, D., & Leitch, I. (2002). Psychotherapy for sexually abused girls: Psychopathological outcome findings and patterns of change. *British Journal of Psychiatry*, *180*(3), 234–247. https://doi.org/10.1192/bjp.180.3.234
Trowell, J. (1988). Child sexual abuse and gender identity development. In D. Di Ceglie (Ed.), *A stranger in my own body: Atypical gender identity development and mental health* (pp. 154–172). Karnac.
Tustin, F. (1990). *The protective shell in children and adults*. Karnac.
Williams, G. (1997). Double deprivation. In *Internal landscapes and foreign bodies* (pp. 33–49). Karnac.
Winnicott, D.W. (1956). Primary maternal preoccupation. In *Collected papers of D.W. Winnicott* (p. 303). Tavistock Publications

In the footsteps of Bick: continuing the legacy of infant observation

Dilys Daws and Alexandra de Rementeria

The authors, both child psychotherapists but from different generations, describe the legacy of Esther Bick in their learning, teaching and clinical practice. In telling two very personal stories about the importance of infant observation in their work, they span 60 years and trace the arc of Bick's legacy over that period.

Introduction

In this paper we, two child psychotherapists from different generations, describe the importance of Bick's method of infant observation in our learning, teaching and clinical practice. In discovering and championing the value of naturalistic observation of infants in their homes, Bick established at least three important factors in developing a psychoanalytic perspective. Firstly, the need to be put in touch with infantile anxieties, secondly, understanding that the trajectory of such anxieties depends largely on the social environment of the infant's family and his relationship to his carers and siblings and, thirdly, that it is in the act of receiving projections and making sense of that experience that the observer learns to work with transferential phenomena.

In telling two very personal stories about the centrality of infant observation in our work, our scope is narrow but the line we trace spans 60 years and does, we hope, sketch the arc of Bick's legacy over that period. There are many detailed and important accounts of the complex and vital ways in which Infant Observation contributes to the training of child and adult psychotherapists and analysts. A good number have been published in this journal (Hinshelwood, 2017, Hopkins, 1994; Likierman, 1997; Crick, 1997), the *International Journal of Psychoanalysis* (Houzel, 2012; Altmann Litvan, 2007, Waddell, 2006; Yakeley, 2017) and the *Journal of Child Psychotherapy* (Daws, 1997; Magagna, 1987; Miller, 1992; Rustin, 1988). The *International Journal of Infant Observation and its Applications* has been charting developments in psychoanalytic observation and its uses in varied professions for more than twenty years and is an invaluable and substantial resource including Margaret Rustin (2009) on Infant Observation in relation to clinical training and Michael Rustin (2006) on Infant Observation as a method of research. We particularly recommend Waddell (2006) and Rustin (2009).

Dilys starts with a personal account of being in Bick's seminar and moves on to comparing notes of observations of two generations of observed infants in one family. We discuss some of the applications of the method in our clinical work and Alex remembers her time in Dilys' observation seminar and then reflects on using the method in her doctoral research and on teaching infant observation in 2021. This paper was given as part of the Tavistock and Portman NHS Trust Centenary Celebrations by Dilys Daws and Alexandra de Rementeria, chaired by Kathryn Fenton.

Dilys

In 1960 I started to train as a Child Psychotherapist at the Tavistock with Juliet Hopkins. The training then took only 3 years, with the first year as the Observation Course. We were on probation that year, and if we passed went on to the 2nd year Clinical Course. The Infant Observation had a first year with Bick and its second year held as the Clinical Course started, was led by Bowlby. His theories were quite different from Bick's. She was more entranced by the internal emotions of the baby, and less concerned by the complex family tensions. Once I explained to him what I felt he was missing out on. I didn't realise how genius-led his theories also were! In 'Child Care and the Growth of Love', already published in 1953 before Juliet Hopkins (Bowlby's niece) and I had started training, he showed how physical proximity in a mother feeding a baby leads to the love that grows between them. This anticipated his later world-influencing work in *Attachment and Loss* (Bowlby, 1969), where he showed how crucial separation is to a child. He emphasised how family relationships affect a child's development and that clinical work with children should include work with their parents. I was lucky to see a child patient, with Bowlby seeing his mother! He had been very helpful to the beginnings of Child Psychotherapy and helped the ACP to be founded, though it had to be named ACP-non-medical, and he continued to give friendly support to the profession. Years later he and I were both giving papers at the 30th Anniversary of the Association of Child Psychology and Psychiatry, now the Association of Child and Adolescent Mental Health (ACAMH). On the platform I was able to apologise to him for my lack of understanding!

Alex, on learning from Dilys

I first met Dilys as a student in her Infant Observation seminar group 15 years ago. I now teach Infant Observation and enjoy telling my students about Dilys telling about being left holding the baby while the parents went to buy curtains during an observation. In particular, that Mrs Bick seemed to understand how that might have happened. I think that this helps them to get a sense of the continuity between Bick and what they are trying to do now but also, that the challenges they face have always been there. But I also tell it to borrow some of Dilys' talent for undercutting any stuffiness that can gather around a method that requires rigour.

I fell pregnant towards the end of my observational studies and Dilys teased me about having done the theory before embarking on the practice. While I was at home up to my ears in practice with a toddler and baby she invited me to help her to update a baby book she had written. During this project I learned more about her generosity and confidence in what might be possible. Once again, Dilys put the importance of observation and her trust in the potential of others at the centre – the book was essentially an invitation to get to know your baby. Rather than guide and advise we described how a parent might come to know all that their baby needed them to know through watching and noticing what happens between them and their baby. Dilys is just the right person to write a baby book because it is only an extension of her clinical work to focus on nurturing the capacity for nurture and containment in the parent. We called it *Finding Your Way with Your Baby* (Daws & de Rementeria, 2021) in an attempt to capture this, that the book was going to help the parent find out who their baby is and what their baby needs, rather than pretend to know from on high. The second edition has just come out.

'Infant observation with Esther Bick' (Dilys)

First to say that it was Alex who thought of the title *Finding Your Way with Your Baby* (Daws & de Rementeria, 2021) for our book. Like my own children she is now one of the new leading creative generation!

Bick's seminars were wonderful. She could be both lovable and terrifying, but the knowledge we gained was inspirational. Soon after I qualified I read her paper 'Notes on Infant Observation in psychoanalytical training' (Bick, 1964). The baby 'James' quoted in this was the one I had observed. She had neither asked me nor told me she was using my notes. Rather different from the policy these days!

I quote from her paper using some of these notes, I think she was actually using the paper I wrote before qualifying, not my weekly notes. In those days the paper was usually a simple story of the observation, not a theoretical one using the notes as examples.

Mrs Bick says:

> Here is a [contrasting] example in which the kinaesthetic pattern is the key to the nature of the relationship. The observation began when baby James was four and a half weeks old. His mother had been undressing him in preparation for the bath as she first put him on his back he tried to reach for the breast and made some

protesting noises, The mother talked to him continually saying "It's horrible isn't it? ... Poor old fellow, never mind, you will soon be in the water". She told the observer that he loved actually being in the water, unlike her other children who disliked it when they were babies. When in the water he lay quietly bringing his knees up to his stomach, making no sound and looking quite contented. In later observations he splashed, kicked and played in the bath and often protested when taken out, as at this first observation when he was four and a half weeks old. When mother put him on to the breast he attached himself to the nipple at once and sucked vigorously. He had his eyes open and with the right hand he touched the breast and the button on the mother's dress alternately. This touching of the mother's body was observed as a regular pattern of behaviour whenever the baby came close to her. At thirteen weeks, the mother gave the observer the baby to hold while she went out to prepare the bath and said "go to your auntie, she's got to study you"; James lay on the observer's lap looking at her, but did not touch her. When the mother returned he looked at her and followed her with his eyes until she took him. On her lap he felt for the breast with mouth and hand and later held her arm with his hand. After the bath, at the breast, he clutched at the breast; his mother removed his hand. He then put his hand on top of the mother's hand and moved it rhythmically while he sucked. At twenty-two weeks he was stroking the breast with wide movements: "At twenty-four weeks (I am quoting from the students notes) James took the breast eagerly. His mother said he would not be having it much longer, the milk was giving out. With his left hand James played with the mother's breast and then with her hand. The movements remained lively all through the taking of the breast. As I watched him I wondered if his movements might be a conscious caressing of the mother; he appeared to me to be aware of what his hand was doing. The mother put James to the second breast and he took this eagerly, stroking her breast and neck and touching her mouth, although usually I have only noticed him do this during the first breast. He was weaned to the bottle at twenty-seven weeks. There followed a week of distress when he refused food, falling asleep between mouthfuls, while sleeping badly at night. The mother remarked that he behaved as though he was a little baby. In the following week he started touching the bottle, later reaching out for it, stroking it lovingly, as he had done with the breast, and eventually settled down to keeping one hand on the bottle and touching, stroking and caressing the mother with the other hand". (Bick, 1964, p. 564)

Esther Bick then says

I have of course described the overall patterns – the gross trends – and have had to omit the many finer details of the ups and downs as time would not permit of recounting them. The material convinced us in the seminar that the relation of this baby to the breast and mother was close and intimate, and he expressed his love as well as anger towards her, predominantly by handling her body. We noted that although the mother was very vocal herself, the baby remained relatively silent with a preference for tactile and kinaesthetic modes of relationship and communication. (Bick, 1964, p. 565)

In this paper Mrs Bick also says:

What we also find is that the students learn to watch and feel before jumping in with theories, and learn to tolerate and appreciate how mothers care for their babies, and find their own solutions. In this way the students are slowly able to

> discard rather fixed notions about right and wrong handling and become more flexible about accepted principles of infant care. What is borne in upon them is the uniqueness of each couple, how each baby develops at its own pace and relates itself to its mother in its own way. (Bick, 1964, p. 565)

This is a key statement of how valuable infant observation is in clinical training for many disciplines, of learning to respect families' relationships and the nature of their problems. Not jumping in with pre-determined solutions, and letting them find their own way.

A few years after I qualified Bick had retired and became ill. I went to visit her at home with my 3 year old son. Although my feeling towards her was mainly respectful, my son was caught up in her charisma. She lay on top of her bed as we talked, and he said 'This is a very nice flat. Could I look round it?' She got off the bed, took his hand, and they walked round it together!

30 years after I did my infant observation a colleague, Kate Steiner, also did an infant observation at the Tavistock, and discovered that the mother of the baby was the sister of my observed baby 'James'! She found this out when the grandmother visited and talked warmly of my observation. The mother then recalled it with some pleasure. Kate got in touch with me, waited until she had finished the observation two years later, and then read my notes, and wrote her dissertation on a comparison of the observations.

One of her themes was how much the two mothers were the same or different. She says 'The study suggests that the repetition of relationship patterns via parents' identification with their own parents is by no means inevitable'. There is also the capacity for growth and change from one generation to another so that 'a mother can repeat some of her experiences of her own mother, but also develop her own style and personality as a mother herself'. She quotes Dinora Pines (1982) 'the representation of an internal mother is a lifelong model for her daughter to identify and also to differentiate from.'

Kate also compares the 2 observations:

> What comes across strongly from this comparison of observations so far apart in time is the sensitivity of the approach and the richness of material that emerge from a study completed when the observational method was in a fairly early stage of development. In fact there are some striking differences in approach in the earlier observation: the visits are recorded in the minutest practical detail with very little personal comment or feeling added; the observer seems more intimately involved with the family than would be advised now, including holding, feeding and bathing the baby(!) and father is noticeably absent in the earlier notes. These differences suggest a fascinating area for further research, but perhaps just as interesting is the sense of continuity provided by Esther Bick's method. I often found it difficult to feel the distance in time between the two families as the richness of observational detail brought the older family so much to life. (unpublished dissertation by Kate Steiner)

Looking myself at my observation notes while writing this paper I was somewhat shocked to see how much I was involved with the baby and family, but I did report all this accurately to Bick and I do not remember ever being criticised for my approach. Perhaps she also enjoyed the interchanges that I reported. As Kate also described the mother of the baby she observed remembering how as children they had all enjoyed reading about themselves in a book I had written (with the parent's consent) as well as hearing anecdotal stories of the observation told by their mother!

It is interesting to think about what Bick chose from my year of observation with her to quote in her paper is James touching of his mother's body, especially her breast, and this on weaning being transferred to his bottle as well as the breast. Bick was one of the earlier people to make the connections so much more common now, between body and mind. A few yeas ago, at an Association of Child Psychotherapy Annual Conference I suggested that in psychoanalytic training, instead of 5 times weekly analysis we should have four times psychotherapy and one session of physiotherapy. Perhaps a more comprehensive way to learn about oneself! This often gets jokingly quoted but hasn't happened yet!

'Infant Observation with Dilys Daws' (Alex)

I find the main challenge in teaching Infant Observation is bringing our attention back to the baby. The group, including me, is always pulled to speculations about the experience of the mother. In a way we contribute to the problem because of our focus on the relational – 'There is no such thing as an infant' we tell them (Winnicott, 1960), then: 'yes, but what about the baby!' when we notice that the baby has slipped out of view. Usually I notice because I get uncomfortable about the hint of judgment creeping in. Wittenberg (1997) tells us that Esther Bick (1964) thought this was a projection into the observer of the mother's own self-doubt and depression. Wittenberg suggests it is also a flight from the horrors of not knowing and from the discomfort of noticing the greed, envy and cruelty that exists alongside the wonderful and the lovely in infants. I tend to agree but I think there is another reason that we are pulled to think more about the internal world of the parents.

As students and teachers of Infant Observation we might suppose that the unconscious is the foreign country that we are trying to get to know. Yet, we seem quite eager, even without much specialist training to speculate about the unconscious motivations of adults. It is the infant's internal world that remains remote. It would seem that Hartley (1953) was right after all – it is the past that is a foreign country. We are inviting students to cross the Rubicon, to transgress the law of infantile amnesia and feel their way, through identification with the closely observed infant, back into their own primitive urges and terrors.

For me, as a student of infant observation, it was in those moments of contact that theories came to life because they applied to me, a part of me I had suddenly accessed through identification with the infant and it was both thrilling and frightening. An experiential, as opposed to theoretical, journey into that other land put me in touch, for the first time, with the fragility of our relationship to reality. I was able to feel again, by proxy, the way that we create as much as discover the world through the distorting prism of our most passionate and primitive impulses. I'd like to share an excerpt from my own infant observation, done under the guidance of Dilys, which helped me understand why none of us can take our relationship to reality for granted.

> The baby is playing with a soft toy mouse-doll and then has a bottle. At around this time his mother was preparing to return to work and was, in various ways, beginning to create some emotional distance between them. It was felt in the seminar group that this was a way of preparing them for, or even an attempt to inoculate them from, the anticipated pain of loss.
>
> *Mum leaves the room to prepare his bottle. The mouse doll is made of a patchwork of brightly coloured fabric. It has enormous long floppy ears and a sausage-like stuffed snout with spindly arms and legs that hang limply. He puts the nose in his mouth. I imagine that it gives a satisfying amount of resistance. He bites harder into it, wrinkling his nose and shutting his eyes with the effort. Taking an ear in each hand, in order to get a better purchase on it, he pulls the mouse away from him and holds the nose fast in his mouth so that he is yanking it so hard in two directions that he starts to wobble. The mouse arms and legs swing violently until eventually he topples over.*
>
> Moments later the feed begins and Mother's role in creating distance during feeding becomes evident, as does his anger about it.
>
> Mother sits cross-legged on the floor opposite me and lifts him into her lap but facing out towards me! She puts the bottle to his mouth and he takes in the teat and sucks and swallows at a fast rate taking half the bottle without a pause. Then he begins to slow the pace and, as he does so, he turns a little so that he is facing side-on and can glance up at her face. He also begins to reach up her body with his left arm so that the back of it gently rubs her breast as he feeds. His face relaxes, as his eyelids flutter and close momentarily. All this is lost when she suddenly props him up again. The arm that had been against her body he now brings round to cup the bottle. Soon he begins to tap the bottle, at first in the distracted and sensual way he had moved his arm up and down her body but increasingly the tapping gets harder and faster until it is more like hitting. He is no longer drinking the milk but holding the bottle in place by biting down on the teat while he hits it from the side
>
> Once his hunger is sated, baby attempts to bring the couple together again through his positioning and caresses. However, when she returns him to his outward-facing disconnected place, the bottle seems to become the recipient of a punitive attack on the withholding mother/breast. Likierman (2001) describes Klein's observation about feeding and weaning: 'When the object becomes available again the infant is simultaneously relieved yet vengeful … these two contradictory impulses are united in the single phantasy of a vengeful devouring.' (p. 104). Baby's play with the mouse-doll seems to betray just such a phantasy. *(8months)* (De Rementeria, 2012, p. 242)

At 8 months this baby might be said to have developed some symbolic functioning. However, this did not feel like 'as if' play. To me it felt that the unprocessed or undischarged devouring urge was awakened by the feeling of the mouse-doll snout in his mouth. He then imbued it with the intention 'withholding' because withholding was the relational antecedent to his sensori-affective state. His world, then, was now home to a withholding mouse, withholding bottle and, despite the displacements, somewhere a withholding mother/breast – all of whom might be expected to be in retaliatory mood after this episode.

I think that Dilys might not agree with all the inferences I make but that I was free to learn deeply from her thinking and allowed to be independent of thought speaks to her generosity of spirit and distaste for theoretical dogma. One of the most important things Dilys gave us was the courage to bear whatever we saw, or thought we saw, no matter how painful. Her power to contain our anxieties meant that we did not have to flinch from pain. When things were hard in a more ordinary way she put things in perspective with her cheerful confidence that all that our infants endured was in the service of freeing themselves for the joys and challenges of their next developmental stage. I think that as a teacher and clinically it is Dilys' hopefulness that is so growth promoting.

Dilys: Teaching of Infant Observation

I have also taught infant observation for many years at the Tavistock, very generously described by Alex who also has added more about the teaching for this paper. I enjoyably saw the development of the trainees, and the seminar group as they described the development of the babies they observed. At the beginning I would point out the importance of finding out where to be in the context of the family, literally where to sit, but how to find their relationship with the family. I found some notes from our seminar with Mrs Bick where I said

> I felt one could use one's clinical judgment to estimate how much the family's behaviour was modified by the presence of an observer, it was usually possible with a little experience to tell what mother and the children were doing because the observer was there and what they would be doing anyhow. Also, there were always times when the mothers were so absorbed in their families that they genuinely seemed oblivious of the observer's presence.

One of the problems for some trainees was in not finding a baby to observe, perhaps more difficult these days because of safe guarding restrictions, but also because of anxiety about the very new experience of observing, recording and presenting to the seminar. I would suggest that they found a baby in a family they knew, friends, family or neighbours, and ask if they could observe it once and discuss it anonymously in the seminar. The experience usually went well. It broke the deadlock and the trainee found a baby very soon. This perhaps also eased their way into clinical work when that started.

Clinical applications

In learning to observe a baby we experience the emotions stirred up by this exposure to the intensity of being with a tiny baby, and the drama of a mother-baby relationship. Learning to observe with respect and with self-containment is a difficult art. It is also a way of learning how to start being a therapist, how to observe what is going on for others in a heightened situation, to note the feelings stirred up in oneself, to learn how to manage them and to use them as a source of information, not as a key to action. We learn to attune to mother and baby and to observe our own feelings.

In psychotherapy we work with emotions, our patients' and our own, and this is most evident when we work with parents and infants. The first duty of parents is to attend to their physical needs – to keep their babies alive. This requires knowledge, skill, instinct and emotionality. How do parents feel about their tiny helpless baby? Where do emotions connect with instincts? How do love and hate fit in to this life and death reality? Are parents developing the love and secure attachment that can grow from the proximity necessary in feeding a baby and keeping it safe? Or are the cues of infantile needs triggering hostility to their baby from parents who feel unable to meet his needs? (Fraiberg et al., 1975).

Our ability to work with parents and infants is drawn from our own experience which remembered or not may lead us to empathise with the situations of others. But human experience is somatic as well as emotional. In parent-infant work bodily realities are everywhere. Babies are fed in front of the clinician, their nappies are changed in the room. These bodily functions and the emotions that accompany them are experienced directly between the baby and his parents. The therapist may be the recipient of transference communications from the parents, but she also observes the parent's perceptions of their baby, influenced by their own past experiences – in other words their transferences on to their baby.

Parents use their emotions to attune appropriately to their newborn baby and his need to be looked after. The feeling of being in touch with each other's emotional state plays a major part in allowing the baby to feel safe enough to 'let go' into sleep. We as therapists are also using our ability to attune to the families we see. We need to be in touch with their state of mind before we can think about how to change it. By knowing their emotional state and then daring to be different we help parents to have the courage to recognize that their infant's state of mind may not be the same as theirs.

The baby in the room

Why do we have the baby in the room? Sometimes there is a remarkable connection between what parents talk about and small babies' actions and vocalizations. Babies are often in tune with the emotional atmosphere and may cry when painful matters are talked about. This can in fact be a clue to why some babies cry excessively; it may connect with some inconsolable experience in the parents' own history. When the parent is able to talk about this with the therapist they may then be able to console the baby (Hopkins, 1994). The parents' reaction to a baby crying in a session may be useful material for the work. Mothers who have difficulty soothing their baby may be trying to do so silently. When I pointed this out to one mother she said 'If I did say anything to him it would be too horrible'. The opportunity to put into words to the therapist the 'horrible' thoughts that she had about the baby came as a release to her. Once some thoughts are said, and acknowledged they may become bearable. A therapist who is non-judgemental can allow parents to own their hostile feelings towards the baby. It enabled the mother to have a different range of feelings towards the baby. She became able to hold him close to her and put into words what he might be feeling. She was no longer preoccupied with the force of her own impulses. The baby sensed this difference and was able to be comforted by his mother's holding of him. The therapist can be thought of as carrying out a symbolic holding of the emotions going around a family; the experience of this holding enables parents to pass it on to their baby.

The therapist must judge consciously or otherwise, to whom to attune to at any moment. She may at times feel attuned to both parent and baby. At other times there is real discordance. I was working with a depressed mother who cried as she talked. Looking at her, with a sympathetic expression, I then found myself looking at her baby who was sitting playing on the floor. He caught my gaze and smiled at me broadly. I smiled at him in return. He was perhaps grateful for an adult who was not crying; he was probably also showing the means he may often have had to use, a smile to cheer up his depressed mother. In any case, I smiled back at him, then looked up again at his mother and was terribly conscious of my incongruent expression, feeling that I had to 'wipe the smile off my face' it was a very useful lesson for me of the dilemma for babies of depressed, mothers – if their mothers cry, will they make things better or worse by smiling?

Silences

I also am interested in how much we therapists talk in these meetings. To teach this style of work in the baby clinic I worked in, I sometimes saw cases jointly with a referring professional, I saw a depressed mother and two hyperactive toddlers with their Health Visitor. The mother cried as she told a story of many losses and the Health visitor put her arm round her. Afterwards the HV and I discussed the meeting. She was impressed with how much the mother had confided in us but then confessed 'At first I couldn't stand the silences. I thought 'What silences?' Compared with a psychoanalytic session it had been all talk!

Silences allow time for thoughts to grow, and time to observe the infant.

Also I believe that professionals of all kinds can extend the scope of their work and be braver. The idea of how much to talk with patients is therefore important. Some of us psychotherapists have learned to talk more, but other workers need to do so less. Instead of offering solutions, 'have you tried such and such?' saying 'tell me more about it.' The idea of free association, of allowing patients the space to follow the line of their own unconscious is difficult. For example, postnatally depressed mothers of infants may, given the chance, relate shocking thoughts of anxiety, anger, self-hatred, hatred to the baby or partner, disturbing dreams and fears of damage that has, or might, happen. There is evidence that a series of meetings with a health visitor can greatly help these mothers. What does hearing this kind of material do to the worker? Anyone who takes on this work needs support and supervision.

The observing stance is the basis for the consultation that is part of what I as a child psychotherapist can offer the baby clinic. At the end of the baby clinic a meeting of health visitors and doctors reviews each attendance, and any worries about the baby and its family are noted. These meetings are a necessary exchange of information and the anxieties accumulated during the two hours or more of the baby clinic. The psychotherapist can be part of the process where anxieties are picked up and highlighted, or where the group reassures itself that it can be left and reconsidered next week. One of my problems was deciding when to help raise the anxiety level in colleagues and when to help settle it. In general practice and in a baby clinic doctors and health visitors are seeing the whole range of the population. In the main they are supporting normality and healthy development. In order for such a clinic to survive there must be a basic assumption that the anxieties brought constantly are being met and dealt with by the routine activities of the clinic. Parents who have just had a baby are normally in a heightened state of emotion; life and death feelings are part of the ordinary state of a baby clinic. Doctors and health visitors have to tolerate the stress of this and evaluate when some of it is out of the ordinary and needs special attention.

The professionals also have to cope with the feelings aroused in themselves. This leads to what may be the most helpful contribution that a psychoanalytically trained worker can bring to a primary care team. This is in helping the team to learn to identify the feelings aroused in them by patients, to help them manage these feelings, and use them as a valuable source of information about feelings the patient may have and be unable to tolerate. I think we learn some of this when we do Infant Observation.

The first paper I wrote about this work was entitled 'Standing by the weighing scales'. The weighing scales are important as a focal part of the baby clinic. The baby's body is looked at measured and appreciated by parents and professionals. Babies' bodies are vulnerable in their nakedness and many mothers intuitively sense this and wrap their babies round with their voice and their gaze as well as with their hands. Others cannot do this and the baby's vulnerability is exposed. All this can be noticed by a receptive health visitor and help her think about what the family needs from her.

It takes as much skill to stand next to a weighing machine as not to talk during a psychotherapy session! The skill of thinking on behalf of a patient is evident if one puts one's thoughts into words, but if one talks too much reflective thought has no time to grow. Standing doing nothing and observing equally requires skill if it is not to be puzzling and persecuting to the people around. It is legitimised in a busy clinic because all professionals stand at times looking around, sometimes deciding what to do next, sometimes talking to each other. I could be any of these, standing to watch what is going on, or ready for discussion. I must be careful not to get annoyingly in the way of busy staff actually trying to weigh the babies, or get to the filing cabinet! If I am too self-contained it must seem that my observations are for some unexplained private use: if I look too efficiently outgoing mothers hand me their baby book to check them into the clinic! By watching I gain what for me is invaluable – seeing a whole range of parents and babies interact. The time I spend is usually a few minutes here and there, between appointments, but weekly my store of information about normality and pathology is reinforced so that when someone is referred to me with a problem, I have a background of knowing where this might fit in with what usually happens between parents and babies.

Clinical applications – Alex

After qualifying as a child psychotherapist I worked in a neurodisability service, involved in diagnosis as well as treatment of children with autism. Adele O'Hanlon, the Psychotherapy Lead in the service articulated that our role was to 'keep uncertainty alive and useful in the context of the pull towards certainty in a diagnostic process.' It was undoubtedly our training in infant observation that enabled us to notice and articulate those moments that confounded attempts at categorising – autistic/ non-autistic. Usually this was to notice where apparently autistic ways of relating might have been adaptive to a particular emotional environment but sometimes it enabled us to see Autistic traits that were being masked by high-functioning children. The use of an adult's hand as a tool is so common as to be thought almost diagnostic in itself. I once worked with a girl who would never have been so concrete but revealed the same difficulty with acknowledging the separateness of the other, of the separateness of her mind as well as body. If she needed help, to find and free the end of the sellotape say, she would not ask for it, nor would she lead my hand to it but she might comment that if we had a piece of sellotape we could mend the paper envelope we were making, while glancing suggestively at the box in which a role of sellotape sat. When a child picks up your hand and places it on a biscuit tin you feel that your personhood has been bypassed and your dexterity is being appropriated rather than requested. In the first scenario there seems to be very little theory of a mind that might command the hand. Yet, it felt almost the same with this little girl, I had been positioned to notice how I might be helpful in such a way that I did not really feel that I had much agency, again my dexterity was being appropriated but through a manipulation of my mind rather than my hand. She knew I had a mind alright, it was the fact that it was my mind and not always 'of a mind' with her mind that troubled her. It was observation, as taught to me by Dilys that helped me to make sense of these experiences and understand the highly nuanced similarities and differences between various forms of neurodisability.

Using infant observation in research

I was also able to indulge my passion for infant observation in my doctoral research. Susan Pawlby at the Bethlem in South London, had been doing research alongside her clinical work at the mother and baby unit there and had a great number of video recorded interactions between mother and baby on admission and discharge archived. She generously made these available to me for my research. There isn't space here to go into that project but I thought it might be interesting to share my first impressions on seeing the videos. Here I try to capture something of the process of applied observation. The initial discomfort of not knowing what you are looking *at* or *for*, followed by a slow coalescing of meaning as one's training in observation makes itself available and the detail of what is seen by and felt by the observer comes together to tell a story.

First impressions

As I watched a dozen or so 3-minute videos I had a range of uncomfortable feelings. The setting and the medium were unfamiliar to me having never used video clinically nor worked in an inpatient setting. I had also never designed a research study and was overwhelmed with a sense of inadequacy to the task. I feared that I would see nothing when I looked at the pairs, that my observation skills would desert me. It had been almost ten years since I'd completed the Infant Observation course as part of my pre-clinical training. To my horror I did not see much at first. Yes, I felt uncomfortable watching the videos but this seemed to have more to do with my own preoccupations than the interactions I watched. About one pair I thought irritably: 'oh for God's sake they seem alright' yet I knew this could not be true. If they were fine they'd be at home. Later I realised that if they had been fine, I would enjoy watching them, but this sort of common-sense understanding was as absent as my capacity for clinical observation. Slowly, as my blunted intellect and sense of panic gave way to something more like boredom, boredom with a deathly quality, I recognised where I was. This unpleasant state of mind was familiar to me from my clinical work doing psychotherapy with very disturbed children. I was emotionally cut-off. However, the more I watched and the more I attuned to my countertransference experience, the clearer it became that this was defensive on my part.

Being in touch with profoundly disturbing infantile anxieties, both those of the baby and those stirred in the mother by her baby, was to become almost intolerable at times during this project but at the beginning I underestimated how powerfully the projections could get into an observer, even through the screen.

Once I'd acknowledged this to myself I began to see much more and I began to see patterns that interested me. One such moment came when I had the opportunity to attend the discharge meeting of a mother and baby whose videos I had seen that morning. In the video mother and baby were struggling to be together. Mother's gaze and voice were intrusive and the baby would often shut her eyes and feign sleep. In response mother would allow her focus to drift away. As baby sensed this she would peek at her mother's face, apparently wanting to take something in from her but only daring to when she was not in danger of catching her mother's eye and interest again. At the pair's discharge meeting I was fascinated to hear the nursery nurse describe how this baby, several months older now, would 'play dead' when she didn't want to comply with what was being asked. With a tone of affectionate chastisement the nurse described noticing a faint smile beneath the baby's closed eyes and slumberous breathing. I was struck by how this defence, one I'd seen develop in response to her mother's intrusiveness, had then gone on to develop into something more playful in relation to adults who were more emotionally available and less frightening.

Much of what we have said in this paper is about putting feelings into words, making our own connections in a way that can make even pe-verbal babies feel understood. But paradoxically silences are just as important, observing and staying with our thoughts and feelings. As the inverted saying goes: 'Don't just do something, stand there'. I hope in our hundredth year, as well as reaching out effectively to many more people, we have retained the importance of a reflective psychoanalytical base for our clinical work and training.

Disclosure statement

No potential conflict of interest was reported by the author(s).

References

Altmann Litvan, M. (2007). Infant observation: A range of questions and challenges for contemporary psychoanalysis. *The International Journal of Psychoanalysis*, *88*(3), 713–733. https://doi.org/10.1516/9031-19R0-3704-2371

Bick, E. (1964). Notes on infant observation in psychoanalytic training. *International Journal of Psychoanalysis*, *45*, 558–566.

Bowlby, J. (1969). *Attachment and Loss, Vol. 1: Attachment*. Basic Books.

Crick, P. (1997). Mother-baby observation: The position of the observer. *Psychoanalytic Psychotherapy*, *11*(3), 245–255. https://doi.org/10.1080/02668739700700211

Daws, D. (1997). The perils of intimacy: Closeness and distance in feeding and weaning. *Journal of Child Psychotherapy*, *23*(2), 179–199. https://doi.org/10.1080/00754179708254541

Daws, D., & de Rementeria, A. (2021). *Finding your way with your baby: The emotional life of parents and babies* (2nd New ed.). Routledge.

de Rementeria, A. (2012). Managing intimacy and distance: An exploration of links between the experience of an observed mother and baby and that of her observer. *Infant Observation*, *15*(3), 231–245. https://doi.org/10.1080/13698036.2012.733516

Fraiberg, S., Adelson, E., & Shapiro, V. (1975). Ghosts in the nursery. A psychoanalytic approach to the problems of impaired infant-mother relationships. *Journal of American Academy of Child Psychiatry*, *14* (3), 387–421. PMID: 1141566. https://doi.org/10.1016/s0002-7138(09)61442-4

Hartley, J. P. (1953). *The go-between*. Hamish Hamilton.

Hinshelwood, R. D. (2017). Infant observation and research: Emotional processes in everyday life. *Psychoanalytic Psychotherapy*, *31*(4), 411–413. https://doi.org/10.1080/02668734.2017.1374044

Hopkins, J. (1994). Therapeutic interventions in infancy: Two contrasting cases of persistent crying. *Psychoanalytic Psychotherapy*, *8*(2), 141–152. https://doi.org/10.1080/02668739400700151

Houzel, D. (2012). Infant observation and the French model. *The International Journal of Psychoanalysis*, *93*(1), 181–201. https://doi.org/10.1111/j.1745-8315.2011.00499.x

Likierman, M. (1997). Psychoanalytic observation in community and primary health care education. *Psychoanalytic Psychotherapy*, *11*(2), 147–157. https://doi.org/10.1080/02668739700700121

Magagna, J. (1987). Three years of infant observation with Mrs. Bick. *Journal of Child Psychotherapy*, *13*(1), 19–39. https://doi.org/10.1080/00754178708254803

Miller, L. (1992). The relation of infant observation to clinical practice in an under fives counselling service. *Journal of Child Psychotherapy*, *18*(1), 19–32. https://doi.org/10.1080/00754179208259361

Pines, D. (1982). The relevance of early psychic development to pregnancy and abortion. *The International Journal of Psychoanalysis*, *63* (3), 311–319. PMID 7129777.

Rustin, M. (1988). Encountering primitive anxieties: Some aspects of infant observation as a preparation for clinical work with children and families. *Journal of Child Psychotherapy*, *14*(2), 15–28. https://doi.org/10.1080/00754178808254824

Rustin, M. (2006). Infant observation research: What have we learned so far? *Infant Observation*, *9*(1), 35–52. https://doi.org/10.1080/13698030600593856

Rustin, M. (2009). Esther Bick: legacy of infant observation at the Tavistock- some reflections 60 years on. *International Journal of Infant Observation and Its Applications*, *12*(1), 29–41. https://doi.org/10.1080/13698030902731691

Waddell, M. (2006). Education section: Infant observation in Britain: The Tavistock approach. *The International Journal of Psychoanalysis*, *87*(4), 1103–1120. https://doi.org/10.1516/195B-8VW0-7287-JVR7

Winnicott, D. (1960). The theory of the parent-infant relationship. *International Journal of Psycho-Analysis*, *41*, 585–595.

Wittenberg, I. (1997). Beginnings: The family, the observer, and the infant observation group. In S. Reid (Ed.), *Developments in infant observation, the Tavistock model* (p. 27). Routledge.

Yakeley, J. (2017). Mind the baby: The role of the nanny in infant observation. *The International Journal of Psychoanalysis*, *98*(6), 1577–1595. https://doi.org/10.1111/1745-8315.12631

Tavistock Centenary: the Tavistock Autism service over four decades

Sue Reid, Anne Alvarez, Nechama Polak and Myooran Canagaratnam

An event held in December 2020 explored the rich clinical work and innovative thinking around Autism Spectrum Condition at the Tavistock over the past four decades. Consultant Child and Adolescent Psychotherapists Sue Reid and Anne Alvarez describe their early groundbreaking work within the Tavistock Autism Team and Workshop. This work yielded the fascinating clinical observations that there were some children with the condition who made significant gains in therapy, leading to major developments in psychoanalytic techniques for this group. Since then, there has been a continuing influence of psychoanalytical, systemic perspectives on the Tavistock approach to Autism. It is an approach which at the same time is firmly rooted in the research around Autism's neurodevelopmental basis. Nechama Polak, Clinical Psychologist, provides an account of how the current work of the team has increasingly focused on supporting young adults with the condition, and their parents, whilst Myooran Canagaratnam, Consultant Psychiatrist, describes the Tavistock approach to diagnostic assessment.

Introduction

This paper is based on a Tavistock and Portman Centenary event held in December 2020, which explored the rich clinical work and innovative thinking around autism spectrum condition at the Tavistock over the past four decades. Consultant Child and Adolescent Psychotherapists Sue Reid and Anne Alvarez describe their early groundbreaking work within the Tavistock Autism Team and Workshop in the 1980s and 1990s. This yielded the fascinating clinical observations that there were some children with the condition who made significant gains in therapy, leading to developments in psychoanalytic techniques for this group. It also provided detailed insights into the nature of the condition and the role of personality in its course. Their work underlined the importance of providing support for parents and siblings, and working with schools and wider networks.

Nechama Polak, Clinical Psychologist and Adult Psychotherapist, who currently works in the service, discusses the role of the service in working with adolescents and young adults with autism over the past 10 years, particularly as they negotiate transitions. Finally, Myooran Canagaratnam, Consultant Child and Adolescent psychiatrist, describes the recent development of the diagnostic service for autism, and how its approach to assessment and post diagnostic work has been influenced by the team's therapeutic roots, as well as contemporary concepts around neurodiversity.

Service origins and developments

Sue Reid

When I started my training, in 1970, I was most fortunate to have the opportunity to work with a child with autism, or to be more accurate, as she was called then, an 'autistic child' (Reid et al., 1981). Thinking back over 50 years really underlines for me the importance of understanding that ideas must develop, and talking about the autism work at the Tavistock, I want to underline that thinking must and should have changed over the years – which is why I thought it important to say that someone was called an 'autistic child or person' and not 'a person with autism'.

At the beginning of my training, I had not even heard of autism and, for many of you, that must be difficult to believe since there are now so many books, articles and so on, by professionals, parents and people with autism.

I was given a post at an educational priority area school to run groups. When I first met the head teacher of the school, a person in fact who had a very strong influence on my development, I was told there was one person who I must put in my groups. This was a little girl, whom I will call Anna, who at that point in time was in the nursery, and whose behaviour – violent outbursts succeeded by complete withdrawal – was a great challenge to everyone. The head feared that they might not be able to keep her, so no pressure there then!

My first sight of Anna had me fascinated. I was greatly supported by her nursery teacher, who gave me a chair to sit on and explained that she would almost certainly take no notice of me. I watched fascinated as this little girl did circuits around the nursery, shaking her hands in front of her and stopping every so often to sniff a child's hair, at which point she would either make an approving 'mmmm' sound or shake her head. Only by close observation could I see that she was in fact circling gradually closer to me, she had noticed my presence. She stopped in front of me, leaned in, and smelled my hair. Fortunately, she gave an approving 'mmmm'. I was careful not to move suddenly and, without turning my head, simply said 'hello Anna'.

At that point, I was very supported by Martha Harris (known as Mattie), head of training from 1960. Her drive was to extend the scope of the child psychoanalytic psychotherapy training within the NHS. When I told her about Anna and that I knew nothing about autism she rather non-committally encouraged me to just find out for myself. But what equipment did I have at this point in time?; two very important things, which I value more and more as the years go by is our training in psychoanalytic infant observation and in young child observation, and the support of my seminar (Reid, 1997). The emphasis in observation is going in with an open mind, not looking for something but discovering what is there to be seen. This has stood me in good stead over the years, I try not to come to the patient with a construct, but to allow the construct to emerge between us.

From infant observation we learn as adults what we discovered as infants; non-verbal communication – gesture, body movement, facial expressions and eyes are the window to the soul.

What else did I learn from my very first contact with someone with autism? Several things: first the importance of the network; Anna's nursery teacher was extraordinarily sensitive, and open to sharing her experiences with me. When I started the group we had many conversations together. What happened in the group impacted on the nursery and vice versa. I also had the support, hard won at first, from the rest of the staff of the school and of the head teacher.

I also discovered that it is essential never to work with a child with autism without being in contact with his or her parents (Alvarez & Reid, 1999; Reid, 1991, 1999a, 1999c). With hindsight I am grateful to the head of the school who insisted that I meet all of the parents of the children in my groups (very unusual in that setting and in those times). She added if they wouldn't come to the school, I had to do a home visit, something for which I had no experience. I did a home visit and it opened a window on the impact on parents of having a child with autism, something I will never forget. Anna's behaviour was so extreme that she had in fact been referred to the local child guidance clinic which was unusual in those days and in this kind of environment. Her parents, however, wouldn't agree at that point, to her attending because they said that it was just for 'mad children'.

Over time, as Anna's behaviour began to change, her parents started coming to the school and pausing to have a chat with me. This led to a shared cooperative journey with parents, with me, with the nursery teacher, and with the school as a whole. Her parents started coming to assemblies and indeed 2 years into our work Anna had a star part in one. All the members of her group were present and we were allowed to sit together rather than in their classroom groups, and one of them, William, shouted *'int' she great, our Anna!'*

Anna discovered 'other children' in a setting which I could ensure was not too overwhelming for her. The other children in the group became incredibly important for her development, and vice versa. They would come to the nursery wall at breaktimes to seek her out and she soon learned all their names and she would constantly ask her teacher 'when coming William, Neville, Wayne … ?' listing the names of the children in her group. Perhaps it would be helpful to say something brief about the other members of the group. William was a 7 year old boy from a large family; his behaviour at home and at school was frequently uncontrollable to the extent that his mother had appealed to the headmistress to have him taken into care (by the end of the group, he was fully embraced within his family). Wayne was a lanky 6 year old boy, who seemed to live within a fantasy world, he had a very strong feeling of his own inadequacy and had no friends. He was delighted to find someone, who as he put it, '*can't do nothing,*' and therefore presented no threat. Neville was a scrawny ten year old, before the new headmistress had taken over, he was actually responsible for running a protection racket in school! His father was in prison and his mother worked as a prostitute. They had a mix of presenting problems, ages, and ethnicities.

I should say here that my previous experience decided me in favour of heterogeneous groups rather than homogenous, and so I tried to get a mix of presenting problems, age and sex. Homogenous groups compete for the identifying symptom, whereas the heterogeneous group offers the child a 'peer group laboratory' in which they can learn about themselves, their impact on others and other's impact on them (Reid & Kolvin, 1993; Reid, 1987, 1993, 1999b).

This first experience helped me really understand that in order to grow we all need roots; we need an environment that supports growth for the inevitable times of drought and hostile conditions. Just as in individual development, so it is in the development of ideas. Opposition came, both from within the psychoanalytic community and without. Within the school, I was initially regarded with some suspicion, being called 'the shrink', but over time, as I had to prove my resilience by spending the first half term as 'relief teacher' and taking playground duty, I was fully embraced by these generous colleagues. In fact, during one half term, two of my colleagues had, with the head teachers support, decorated a room at the top of the school so as to provide an appropriate environment for psychotherapy groups.

Well, what else did I learn; I learned that the world of the child with autism is 'a world apart.' (A. Reid, 1990). And often a cause of considerable distress to their parents and to their siblings. There's not enough space within this paper to develop those ideas further here. I also discovered that I had to learn to 'walk' in each child's shoes because, each child with autism is unique, so no prescriptive intervention can be effective. I had to mobilise all my curiosity: why does he or she do this? Why won't he or she do that? How do they experience me and the world around them? When, and under what conditions, do they seem to function most optimally and what conditions impact upon them adversely?

My early experience with Anna taught me to rely on my own experience and have the courage of my convictions, whilst being open to the ideas of others. Essential for me in learning to be resilient. I did not know that many people held the view that children with autism could not change. I learned from my own experience that indeed, sometimes they could.

When I qualified Mattie Harris continued to be a support and suggested that any referrals of children with autism should come to me. What started as a slow trickle, gradually gathered pace by word of mouth; one family encouraging another family to try us and schools who found a child seemed to benefit from the contact with us, encouraging other parents also to give us a try.

One day, in the early 80s, I realized I was supervising 7 trainee child psychotherapists who were working with children with autism. I began to see patterns in their behaviour, aware of the importance of adapting my way of working from the more classical psychoanalytic approach. I was encouraged to set up a seminar and I will be forever grateful for this opportunity. Here I must mention my colleague Trudy Klauber, who joined us as a newly qualified child psychotherapist. She contributed not only her keen intelligence, but was also generous enough to take minutes of our meetings. This has allowed us to track our thinking as it has developed over the years.

In 1986, I founded the autism research workshop and the Tavistock autism service. We were joined by many colleagues who have made major contributions to thinking about autism, and here I should mention especially Maria Rhode (consultant child and adolescent child psychotherapist), Anthony Lee (research psychologist, who also trained as a child psychotherapist) and of course Anne Alvarez – whose work is known to many of you and who became co-convener of the workshop. Anne will be describing many of the further developments in our thinking. The workshop was initially open to people training in the Tavistock but then we were joined by people from around the country and then by colleagues from abroad, contributing to a lively exchange of ideas.

The work was supported particularly by Dr Caroline Lyndsey, psychiatrist and chair of the department, and by many generous colleagues outside, and here I must mention Theresa Wasilewska (educational psychologist) and Johanna Rugieri (headteacher). The Tavistock was purely NHS funded in those days, which made it possible to travel around Britain, sharing our findings with others and also to take referrals from around the country. Within the workshop, there was a lively, creative atmosphere which allowed for 'playing with ideas' and we were free to think together about the technical adjustments we had to make if we were really to reach these children (please see further publications by myself and colleagues mentioned here). These were based on detailed presentations of the children's sessions.

As an NHS department we were, quite rightly, expected to respond to anyone who was referred to us, and this meant we had access to children of all ages from the very young to older adolescents. One important discovery was that the earlier we could intervene, the more profound the impact was likely to be on the child's development.

However, when some of the children showed signs of improvement, we were sometimes told that they must have been misdiagnosed in the first place. We were encouraged initially by Albert Reid, Specialist Psychologist, to video our case studies (our systemic family therapist colleagues were already using video). This generated a number of research projects with Dr Lee measuring the impact before, during, and after treatment. Anne will describe this further.

There were so many developments over the years, but the one I feel most pleased about was the increasing involvement of our patient's parents. I formed a group for the parents of the children in treatment, together with Trudy Klauber, and some of these parents generously gave of their time in organising a series of conferences beginning in 2003, at which they and our patients were speakers. Our patient's trust in us and their generosity, supported all of our work. And here I would say that contact with these parents made so clear that autism is no respecter of social background, ethnicity or religion, it can occur in any family.

Anne Alvarez

I had my first taste of working with children with Autism in Canada in 1962 just before I started my training at the Tavistock. Later, I stopped working at the Tavistock for about 14 years while I was raising my children – working only privately although I still taught on the Tavistock child psychotherapy training. When I came back in the late 80s, Sue and I were both supervising a trainee, Janet Bungener, and she kept telling us that we were saying similar things about technique with children with autism, and the ways it might differ from classical psychoanalysis. Eventually, we got together with her to discuss a patient and found that indeed she was right. I remember us also talking about the fact we had both been discussing the problem of perspective for these children but we were talking about two different versions of perspectives: which angle you look at something from, versus how far away it is. Sue then invited me to join her as co-chair of the Autism Workshop.

Another similarity that emerged was to do with the introduction of a more intensified response to what we both saw as the emptiness in some children with autism. This involved a recognition that some of these children had a genuine deficit in interest in, or desire for, other people, or the world. I had on one occasion found myself in a state of terrible urgency about the nearness of my patient Robbie to a kind of psychic death. I had stopped work for a few months to have a baby, his mother had had a baby during the same period, and I was now only seeing him once a month. I felt I was losing him for good. On this day, the last session before a 2 month summer break, I got increasingly alarmed, and eventually responded with great urgency to how far gone he seemed. I put my face in his line of vision, calling his name over and over. He had seemed to awaken from a deep sleep or a deep drowning and greeted me with a kind of slow delighted surprise – as though he hadn't seen me for a very long time. He said Hello-o- o. He then, the next day, had a breakdown or breakout from his autism and sobbed for a week telling his parents about a trauma he had had, indeed the whole family had had, when he was 2. I then spent years wondering what I had done in that session, as it seemed pretty un-psychoanalytic. It wasn't neutral, but nor was it even containing, to use the then more modern terminology of Bick (1968) and Bion (1962). I eventually termed it a kind of reclamation; others have pointed out it is a kind of vitalization (Alvarez, 1980, 1992), (Director, 2009). I came to conclude that Robbie was not hiding, he was lost, he was not withdrawn, he was undrawn. His apparent emptiness was not due to resistance, he really had become empty.

During the same period, it turned out that Sue was making a similar discovery. She was identifying something she was doing to show her autistic patients that the world could be interesting, namely a 'generation' and a 'demonstration' of the value and interestingness of the world – of toys or objects in the room (S. Reid, personal communication, 1988). She was careful, however, when I got over-enthusiastic about vitalization to point out that these more intensified methods could be counter- productive with another type of child with autism, those who can easily feel very intruded upon and are more avoidant. We began to be interested in sub-groups (Alvarez & Reid, 1999). I think we took great comfort from the fact that the other was also trying to find new ways of addressing the nature of the disorder when the classical psychoanalytic methods didn't seem adequate. We came to say that the work with these children needed to be not only psychoanalytically informed ie working in the relationship, but also developmentally informed and psychopathologically informed.

Developmentally informed, because the non-autistic part of the personality, often hidden behind the autism, was often very developmentally delayed compared to the child's actual chronological age. Another patient of mine, Samuel, was 3 years old, but his score – on the Vineland Adaptive Behaviour Scale of expressive communication skills – lay at the profoundly low level of 1 month of age. The gap is not always as dramatic as that, but nevertheless, it can be easy for people to confuse this immaturity with the autism itself.

The second thing that was preoccupying to us both was the problem of how to deal with the autistic, repetitive – often relentlessly repetitive – behaviours and interests. Ordinary interpretations and explanations were often not effective when the child was being almost hypnotized by his own bad habits of mind. We were both finding a variety of ways of approaching these, e.g. sometimes actively discouraging, sometimes trying to join in with a bit of accompaniment, e.g. tapping feet in the same rhythm just to get noticed a bit. Again, this was not pure classical analysis meant to encourage reflection. We were both aware that these were not symbolically meaningful activities: I called them addictive, Sue said the child was sometimes simply very stuck. What we both wanted to do was find a way to clear a little space in the child' s mind for something new to enter, and it was not easy. Indeed, Sue has written about the importance of building a mind (Reid, 2019).

A third problem that concerned us, again following from the particular nature of the autistic condition, is that when we did manage to succeed in attracting the child's attention away from his ritual, he seemed to have no idea what else could be available. In this respect, his lack of resources resembled that of neglected children, but for different reasons. We found that if we left the child to his own devices for that moment he just returned to the repetitions. We had to, very quickly, offer something else, hopefully enticing enough to grab and hold his attention. I called it being a bit like a traffic policeman, Sue called it conducting the orchestra, encouraging the string section for example.

Sue has said that when kids did well in our treatment, people often said well they couldn't have been autistic in the first place. We were keen to do some research with before and after measures – I went to see our Professor Izzie Kolvin who suggested a single-case study with the treatment videoed. I then did a 4 year study with Tony Lee, a research psychologist who had joined our workshop, and who later went on to train as a child psychotherapist. In the meantime, he helped both of us and many other people at the Tavistock to design our studies. He and I developed a series of scales for measuring the child's relatedness or lack of it, and were able to show considerable improvements. We measured changes in the number of times the child looked at me, and the duration of his glances. We had raters rate whether the glances were odd or direct. That simplification nearly broke my clinician's heart because Tony insisted we had no space to distinguish between the different types of odd look. But, for a clinician, nuance is everything!!! We also measured Samuel's emotional engagement and level of interest (Alvarez & Lee, 2004). That study was published, and at present we are waiting to resume the writing up of a second study where we developed a different rating scale-one, that measured the kind of interpretation I was making at particular points in time. It shows that over time I moved up a level from a more intensified reclaiming vitalizing level to a more descriptive level which we think suggests the child was becoming more accessible and reachable. The scale was developed with Tony and Vije Franchi, a Tavistock trained child psychotherapist who was Assistant Professor at the University of Geneva. The scale was based on a schema I had suggested for thinking about three different levels of intervention with patients ranging from being in mild neurotic states through borderline, to more autistic or even psychotic or dissociated states of mind (Alvarez, 2012). I would love someday if I live long enough to go back and look at those looks, and also to notice the effects of the 'wrong' level of interpretation on Samuel as opposed to when I got it right. He was not able to say so verbally but he certainly showed me when I got it wrong – he just retreated from a moment of contact to return to his autistic behaviours. Sue and I still work together but I'm sure we both still miss that workshop – it was an exciting time.

Building bridges: working therapeutically with adolescents and young adults

Nechama Polak

Building bridges is essential to any therapeutic task but is particularly relevant to the work of the Autism spectrum disorder and Learning Disability (ASD and LD) team. Celebrating the centenary of the Tavistock Centre, we build a bridge between the legacy of the past and the present in the context of organisational changes and commissioning. We are also creating a bridge for a whole new client population which did not have access to psychotherapy in the past, namely older adolescents and younger adults with autism spectrum condition. Transitioning into secondary school and into adulthood is an important bridge we are creating. Other more obvious bridges are between the external and the internal world, between a child/young person on the spectrum and his family, a child/young person and his therapist and a child/young person and his network/ broader environment. Last but not least we are creating a bridge between the different modalities of work and different clinicians in the team.

A word which is often being used in therapeutic work with children and young people on the spectrum and with learning disabilities is 'adaptation'. Do we adapt the work and if so, how do we adapt? One can say we adapt with every single patient we see as every person is different. There are also no two people on the autistic spectrum who are similar, so adaptation is part of the therapist–patient relationship. We do find though that some general adaptations happen with many patients on the spectrum. On many occasions we would find ourselves reaching out more, being more active as therapists in terms of our stance, though this may vary a lot. The focus of the work for young people can be emotional regulation, identity, understanding themselves better, understanding others and their responses to them as well as managing their difficult emotions as social interactions can be painful and frustrating. In the literature some may call it mentalising and developing of a theory of mind.

The ability to generalise learning and change is something which is debatable in our client population. Can our patients generalise from one relationship to the other, from one setting to the other or from one situation to the other? In my EMDR work with children and young people on the spectrum I have learned that we often need to process every single 'trauma' that happened as the ability to generalise from one situation to another is often quite minimal. That puts a big question mark on the ability for learning. However, a child who was bullied still deserves some processing of their trauma even if it doesn't necessarily decrease the chance of them being bullied again.

We often encounter limitations in the ability to relate and think which demands creativity on the therapist side. Such an environment of continuous impaired abilities can also have a strong impact on our ability as therapists to relate and think and poses a huge challenge to our team. We can often find ourselves doubting our own abilities to help our patients developing these skills.

Which brings me to one of the biggest questions we and our patients deal with in the work; What are the expectations of the work/or what is the 'task' of therapy? There are some bridges we could create but there are some which are more difficult to cross. In our work, it is also important to recognise what we cannot do and help our patients and their families to accept it and mourn it.

Thinking of the current work of our team and the complexity of the referrals we are receiving, it is important to be able to keep a realistic position of what it is that we can achieve. We often see adolescents and young adults who have profound challenges and who would need a lifelong support, which our team will not be able to offer. However, the wish that we could and the push for it, from patients, services and ourselves is strong. We cannot see every child and young person on the spectrum in Greater London and even more so, we cannot be the only ones who are in charge of their care. We often get referrals of cases that have been involved with many services and come to us as a last resort. Like many other services nowadays our waiting list is long, and patients and families can find themselves waiting while experiencing huge distress and challenges. The pressure can at times compromise our ability to serve as a container to these struggling patients and families. Often other services drop, disappear very soon after a referral was made and we can be left in a helpless lonely place, a feeling which may represent how many of our families are feeling.

Young People we see often state that the world needs to adapt to them and not them needing to try and 'fit' into the world. Many young people claim that they are happy with the way they are, whereas their system, their families, really struggle. I recall seeing a woman who presented with an extreme sensitivity to light. She used to walk into the therapy room and switch the lights off straight away without asking if I am ok with it. I saw her for an assessment for group work and the issue escalated when she joined a group of 5 others who didn't wish to sit in the dark. This raised different questions: is it 'only' a sensitivity to light and everyone should sit in the dark, or does it represent an over sensitivity to the world and a lack of ability to fit in? or all the above. Does anyone else need to fit in and sit in the dark and how do you consider individual differences in a group, how do you relate to the other? How do you negotiate it? Do these young people really not feel that they struggle and only others need to manage life with them? These dilemmas are there in our work in individual psychotherapy, psychoeducation, cognitive behavioural therapy, parent work and group work in our team. We offer support for children and young people themselves, to their families and in recent times more and more support to parents either in the couple or in the form of parents group. Many of our families can feel isolated in their struggles and a bridge between parents, either in the couple or with other parents can offer crucial and priceless support.

A therapeutic approach to diagnostic assessment

Myooran Canagaratnam

The autism service at the Tavistock was founded as an innovative psychotherapeutic treatment service. Over the last 10 years a significant development has been the establishment of a diagnostic assessment clinic within the team. This development has occurred in response to an increasing demand for assessments for adolescents and young people of relatively high cognitive functioning. There have been many reasons proposed for this rise in demand – including increasing awareness of the condition, extension of the diagnostic boundaries, and also a recognition that females with the condition may have been underidentified due to differences in their presentation (Skuse, 2020). In our clinical practice, we are also acutely aware of the increasing social pressures young people face, as well as the constraints on resources for supporting them in school, driving a wish to formalise their needs with a diagnostic label.

The fact that the clinic evolved within a psychotherapeutic treatment service has influenced its distinctive approach to the task of diagnosis. The National Institute for Health and Care Excellence (NICE, 2011) recommended approach to diagnostic assessment entails careful collection of information from parents, the young person, and their educational setting regarding the young person's current and historic impairments in social communication and restricted, repetitive behaviour and sensory issues. These processes and assessments are predicated on the condition's well-established neurobiological/organic basis, and at a psychological level, cognitive theories – for example that people with autism have deficits/delays in theory of mind (Happe & Frith, 1995). In our service we follow these processes, using standardised diagnostic assessment tools such as the Autism Diagnostic Observation Schedule, Second Edition (Lord et al., 2012) to help us make a diagnosis – as well of course as the accumulated experience of educational and clinical psychologists, social workers, speech and language therapists and psychiatrists.

At the same time our approach to assessment process draws on the psychoanalytic (Alvarez & Reid, 1999; Hobson, 2014), and systemic (Simon et al., 2020) and attachment (Bowlby, 1969) theories, which are part of the DNA of both the service and the Tavistock Clinic. This breadth of perspectives helps make sense of puzzling aspects of the condition – the heterogeneity of its presentation in different individuals, the associated psychological issues and psychiatric disorders that frequently accompany it, the presence of autistic symptoms in the non-autistic population, and their high incidence in specific groups such as severely maltreated children (Rutter et al., 2007). It also sheds light on the mutability in the condition's features observed over time and across contexts. Sue Reid, above, contrasts the commonly held view in the 1980s that children with autism cannot change, to her own experience from long-term therapeutic work with these children. The differing trajectories of children with autism also fits with our experience gathering information on the early history of the adolescents we see for diagnosis. The degree and nature of change appears highly variable however, which offers both hope, fear and uncertainty for families. Such conflicting feelings may also be experienced by young people and families during the process of diagnosis itself, which can often take several years. We see the role of the clinician is as much accompanying the family on this journey as collecting the required information to reach its conclusion.

Diagnostic assessment of adolescents and young adults raises some particular issues, to which the cross fertilisation of ideas from different disciplines can be brought to bear. Firstly, there is the question of consent. Sometimes of course it is young people themselves who seek referral – increasingly aware of their difference to their peers. Quite often it is parent(s), teachers or other professionals. We have increasingly realised the importance of spending some time at the outset clarifying who is asking for this assessment, and for what purpose. What does the young person themself understand about autism? What might a diagnosis mean for them, what might be its benefits or drawbacks. Some young people may not want what they perceive as a stigmatising label marking them out as 'different'. Others feel it helps them understand themselves better, and provides some validation of their experience. And probably most of them aren't sure either way. This can be difficult for parents who have often battled for a long time for a referral, though parents themselves are often also ambivalent about diagnosis.

Sometimes we might conclude that the issues young people referred are experiencing are not actually due to autism, but have another origin – including mental health difficulties such as depression, anxiety or other developmental issues such as attention deficit hyperactivity disorder. Or we might view the issues they have in social relationships and rigidity as due to the developmental impact of early adverse experiences and trauma. Most commonly, however there is a complex interaction between what Anne Alvarez refered to as the 'autistic' and 'non autistic' aspects of their personality, their environment and of course their experience. As an experienced Child Psychotherapist once said to me 'We don't always see the Autism ... we see the young person's response to it'. We observe a variety of responses to Autism and the difficult experiences of peer rejection, isolation and the sense of being overwhelmed which are often associated with it. Some of these responses can be understood in terms of defence mechanisms. such as withdrawal into autistic fantasy, displacement, acting out, and projection (Freud, 1936). These lead to further pushing social contact away with consequent effects on psychological development.

But there is also the potential for the individual to harness their strengths of personality to engage with the real world (Alvarez & Reid, 1999), and find their place within it. Fundamental to the psychotherapeutic work Alvarez and Reid have described is an appreciation of the individuality of each person with ASC and attention to their context. We endeavour to approach diagnosis in this spirit, though it necessarily takes place over just a few contacts. In addition to behavioural reports and standardised observations, we meet with young people individually, with an aim of more broadly understanding their experience of the world and relationships, and something of their strengths. We have found projective assessments, which allow free-flowing responses to the presentation of a stimulus (Kennedy et al., 2017), particularly useful in this regard. For example, in the Kinetic Family Drawing (Burns & Kaufman, 1970), the child or young person is given blank white paper and pencils and asked to draw everyone in their family, including themselves, doing something. They are asked to draw whole people, not cartoons or stick figures and no time limit is set. Once the drawing is finished, the client is asked to identify each figure, to describe their actions, with further follow-up enquiry (Kennedy et al., 2020). This allows exploration of the young person's view of themselves in the context of the family, and family relationships/dynamics. Another assessment, which we commonly use, is the Sentence Completion Task, consisting of initial phrases, called stems, that young people are asked to extend into complete sentences. Stems may vary in length and structure from just one or two words (e.g., If only ...) through to more detailed statements (e.g., Students in my class ...) Responses are analysed for themes generating hypotheses regarding beliefs, motivations and values (Kennedy et al., 2020).

We also meet with young people with their families to explore how their symptoms impact them, what has been the meaning ascribed to them, and explore impact of culture and ethnicity. School visits and consultations provide information on another important context that young people navigate. Young people are coming to us at a time of their lives when they are experiencing acute pressure from several sources – peer relationships are becoming increasingly complicated, they are negotiating the hurdles of exams, and they are faced with what might happen after they finish school

More generally adolescence is a time where young people are grappling with issues of identity (Waddell, 2018). We are very mindful of the impact a diagnosis can have at this sensitive time. The concept of neurodiversity (Singer, 1999) has influenced the way we think about autism spectrum condition in terms of difference rather than a disorder, albeit a difference that can bring many challenges, but also strengths. The world tends to be organised according to the needs of neurotypical people. We hope that by identifying autism spectrum condition through the diagnostic process, we can empower young people with greater self knowledge. But we also hope it is the spur for those around them to make the necessary changes to promote inclusivity. In this way, those with ASC can achieve the potential they have to make valuable contributions to the community and live fulfilling lives.

Trainees in our service make a great contribution to delivery and development. I wanted to end with an excerpt from a letter a trainee educational psychologist wrote to a young person she worked with, because I think it encapsulates how we think about autism, personality, development and uncertainty:

> One important thing you shared was that the diagnosis from the ASC team had been useful, and that it had been like a piece of a jigsaw to help you to understand one aspect of yourself. I would like to encourage you to keep finding the metaphorical jigsaw pieces, but also to recognise that this is a life-long task, and that everyone is still developing and changing.

Disclosure statement

No potential conflict of interest was reported by the author(s).

References

Alvarez, A., & Lee, A. (2004). Early forms of relatedness in autism. *Clinical Child Psychology and Psychiatry*, *9*(4), 499–518. https://doi.org/10.1177/1359104504046156

Alvarez, A., & Reid, S. (1999). *Autism and personality: Findings from the Tavistock Autism workshop*. Routledge.

Alvarez, A. (1980). Two regenerative situations in autism: Reclamation and becoming vertebrate. *Journal of Child Psychotherapy*, *16*(1), 69–80. https://doi.org/10.1080/00754178008255009

Alvarez, A. (1992). *Live company: Psychoanalytic psychotherapy with autistic, borderline, deprived and abused children*. Routledge.

Alvarez, A. (2012). *The thinking heart: Three levels of psychoanalytic therapy with disturbed children*. Routledge.

Bick, E. (1968). The experience of the skin in early object-relations. *International Journal of Psychoanalysis*, *49*(2), 484–486.

Bion. (1962). *Learning from experience*. Heinemann.

Bowlby, J. (1969). *Attachment and loss, Vol. 1: Attachment*. Hogarth Press and Institute of Psycho-Analysis.

Burns, R. C., & Kaufman, S. H. (1970). *Kinetic family drawings (K-F-D): An introduction to understanding children through kinetic drawings*. Brunner/Mazel.

Director, L. (2009). The enlivening object. *Contemporary Psychoanalysis*, *45*(1), 121–139. https://doi.org/10.1080/00107530.2009.10745990

Freud, A. (1936). *The ego and the mechanisms of defence*. Hogarth Press and the Institute of Psycho-Analysis.

Happe, F., & Frith, U. (1995). Theory of mind in autism. In E. Schopler & G. B. Mesibov (Eds.), *Learning and cognition in autism* (pp. 177–197). Springer.

Hobson, R. P. (2014). The coherence of autism. *Autism*, *18*(1), 6–16. https://doi.org/10.1177/1362361313497538

Kennedy, E. K., Canagaratnam, M., & Shaldon, C. (2017). The use of projective assessment with children and young people. *Assessment & Development Matters*, *9*(2), 25–28.

Kennedy, E.-K., Blyth, F., Sakata, E., Yahyaoui, L., Canagaratnam, M., & Nijabat, K. (2020). Making meaning from experience: Collaborative assessment with young adults who have mental health needs and social communication differences. *Educational & Child Psychology*, *37*(3), 86–98.

Lord, C., Rutter, M., DiLavore, P., Risi, S., Gotham, K., & Bishop, S. (2012). *Autism diagnostic observation schedule–2nd edition (ADOS-2)*. Western Psychological Services.

NICE. *Autism spectrum disorder in under 19s: Recognition, referral and diagnosis, clinical guideline [CG128]*. Retrieved September, 2011 from https://www.nice.org.uk/guidance/cg128

Reid, S. (1987). The use of groups for therapeutic interventions. *Educational and Child Psychology*, *4*(3/4), 171–179.

Reid, A. (1990). *Autism a world apart*. Channel Four Television.

Reid, S. (1991). Group work with children in schools. In M. Fox, and L. Kennedy (Eds.), *Proceedings of the 1991 Conference for Educational psychologists in training*. Tavistock Clinic.

Reid, S. (1993). Group psychotherapy for children and adolescents. In M. Garralda (Ed.), *Managing children with psychiatric problems*. BMJ.

Reid, S. (1997). *Developments in infant observation: The Tavistock model*. Routledge.

Reid, S. (1999a). The assessment of the child with autism: A family perspective. *Clinical Child Psychology and Psychiatry*, *4*(1), 63–78. doi:10.1177/1359104599004001006

Reid, S. (1999b). The group as a healing whole: Group psychotherapy with children and adolescents. In M. Lanyado & A. Horne (Eds.), *The handbook of child and adolescent psychotherapy: Psychoanalytic approaches*. Routledge.

Reid, S. (1999c). The assessment of the child with autism: A family perspective. In A. Alvarez, and S. Reid (Eds.), *Autism and personality: Findings from the Tavistock Autism workshop* (pp. 13-32). Routledge.

Reid, S. (2019) *Building a mind* [Paper presentation]. Developmental Psychology in the Clinic and Beyond Conference, Haifa, Israel.

Reid, S., Fry, E., & Rhode, M. (1981). Working with small groups of children in primary schools. In M. Boston, and D. Daws (Eds.), *The child psychotherapist and problems of young people* (pp, 31-62). Wildwood House.

Reid, S., & Kolvin, I. (1993). Group psychotherapy for children and adolescents. *Archives of Diseases in Childhood*, *69*(2), 244–250. https://doi.org/10.1136/adc.69.2.244

Rutter, M., Kreppner, J., Croft, C., Murin, M., Colvert, E., Beckett, C., Castle, J., & Sonuga-Barke, E. (2007). Early adolescent outcomes of institutionally deprived and non-deprived adoptees. III. Quasi-autism. *Journal of Child Psychology and Psychiatry*, *48*(12), 1200–1207. PMID. 18093025. https://doi.org/10.1111/j.1469-7610.2007.01792.x

Simon, G., Evans, M., Cano, F., Helps, S., & Vlam, I. (2020). Autism and systemic family therapy. In K. S. Wampler, M. Rastogi, and R. Singh (Eds.), *The handbook of systemic family therapy* (pp. 407-432). Wiley.

Singer, J. (1999). Why can't you be normal for once in your life?: From a "Problem with No Name" to a new category of disability. In M. Corker, and S. French (Eds.), *Disability discourse* (pp. 57-67). Open University Press UK.

Skuse, D. (2020). Autism – 25 years on: A lot has changed! *Clinical Child Psychology and Psychiatry*, *25*(3), 721–725. https://doi.org/10.1177/1359104520929729

Waddell, M. (2018). *On adolescence* (1st ed.). Routledge. https://doi.org/10.4324/9780429437458

Shapes of gender identity: three stories with impact

Domenico Di Ceglie

The paper describes three stories of children and adolescents with atypical gender identity development followed in psychotherapy. These cases have already been published, but are revisited here to show how these experiences contributed to the creation of the therapeutic intervention model of the Gender Identity Development Service originally established in 1989 at St George's Hospital, London. The service transferred to the Tavistock Centre in 1996. The first case shows the gradual recognition of dealing with the development of an atypical gender identity rather than a psychiatric condition. Reflection on this case led to the definition of possible therapeutic goals. The second case illustrates the difference between solid and fluid identities, an important distinction in the decision to consider the possibility of physical intervention. The third case shows the network management model and addresses issues concerning autonomy.

Introduction

This presentation, which was given at the Tavistock Centre via Zoom on the 16th of February 2021, describes the early history and origins of the Gender Identity Development Service (GIDS) and of its model of care and philosophy.

Within the Centenary Events of the Tavistock, it seems particularly appropriate to reflect on the foundations of a service which has a focus on the complex dynamics of identity development and, in particular, of gender identity.

I will do this by briefly describing three cases which made a significant contribution to the construction of the original model through the use of 'observation and imagination' in the words of Donald Meltzer as well as of clinical experience and available empirical research.

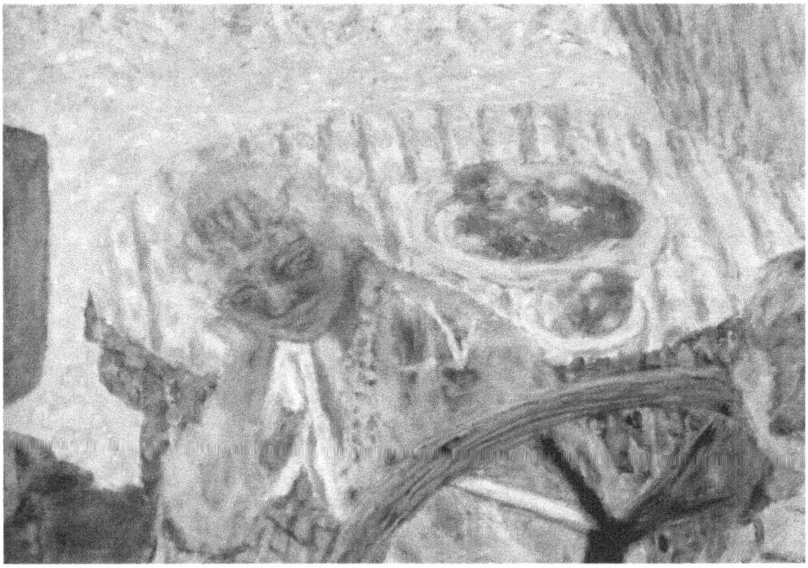

Figure 1. *Young women in the garden* by Pierre Bonnard.

> *Young Women in the Garden* [Figure 1] is one of the most extreme examples of a painting made over a long period of time. Having started work in 1921–3, Bonnard put the canvas aside for many years before revisiting and revising it in 1945–6. Resuming his work was part of an attempt to rediscover the original experience, bringing it into the present without losing its place in the past. (Matthew Gale, curator of the exhibition 23 Jan-6 May 2019, Tate Modern)

In this presentation, I will use a similar approach to that of Bonnard to three cases that I saw in the past and published. I will look at these cases from a new perspective applied to the case material: their impact in the creation of a model of care for children and adolescents with atypical gender identity development or gender diversity, in today's language.

Case 1

Jennifer was 16 when she was referred in the eighties to the Adolescent Department of Tavistock Clinic following three suicide attempts. She had been assigned female at birth, but perceived herself as a male. She presented very distressed with depressive episodes and a number of features which at the time were considered borderline. Today we would have looked more closely for the presence of autistic spectrum features as she had difficulties in communication and avoided eye contact. Recent studies have shown the presence of autistic spectrum features in some transgender people (Di Ceglie et al., 2014; Jones et al., 2012; Skagerberg et al., 2015). A large part of the session was spent in silence. At the time of the referral, Jennifer was still living in a female role, maintained her female name and wished to be addressed using a female pronoun. She was uncertain about physical interventions. Her mother, who had died just before Jennifer came to the clinic, had suffered depression after Jennifer's birth, and her father had been physically violent towards his wife during Jennifer's childhood, until they separated. During her psychotherapy sessions she remembered episodes when her father, in fits of temper, had kicked her mother in the stomach. In one session she admitted, not without a sense of embarrassment and shame, that she had identified with him, an experience that she could not explain. She loved her mother, and her main aim in life was to do something extraordinary that would have made her mother happy. There was no recollection that Jennifer herself had been physically abused by her father, but witnessing violence between her parents had been a traumatic childhood experience.

It is possible to hypothesize that the way Jennifer coped with the fear of damage to her mother, and possibly to herself, was to identify with a male, possessing the strength of a masculine body. Once established, this gave her a sense of survival and also a sense of protecting in her mind the 'damaged' mother. A female representation of herself had to be strongly avoided, as it was equated in her mind with being weak and damaged.

Another important factor also seemed to play a part. After the birth of two older sisters, her mother had miscarried a baby boy. One year later, Jennifer was born. Jennifer seemed to feel that her mother had expected her to be a boy, and in one session she alluded to her mother having 'psychic qualities', as if she had been part of a magical experience in which she and her mother could read each other's mind. She had probably received, and made her own, her mother's wish that she had been a boy. Her mother probably never consciously expressed this wish, but possibly it remained unconsciously active in the relationship between them.

Two years of psychotherapeutic exploration with this young person allowed the therapist, together with Jennifer, to make this partial reconstruction of her childhood relating to her atypical gender identity development. However, any attempts to explore this understanding further with Jennifer led to continuous interruptions of the therapeutic work, which may have indicated her extreme resistance and fears of having the foundation of her gender identity revisited.

Even if Jennifer retained some of this understanding, it certainly did not alter her gender identity development, that is to say, the sense of who he was. His male gender identity seemed well established and fixed. It formed very early in life, and it is likely that traumatic events had played some part in it.

Towards the end of therapy, Jennifer was able to live in a male role with a male name and his well-being improved. He did not attempt suicide again. He settled in a job and he was more able to establish relationships with other people. One might say that therapy had helped him to cope with his well-established gender identity in a better way, to make the transition to a male role and to give him a sense of hope (an important therapeutic aim). He was eventually referred to an adult gender identity service to explore further his perceived identity and the distress generated by the incongruence between his perceived gender and his sexual body. Physical interventions, aimed at harmonizing his gender identity and his body, could also be considered in the adult service.

I became aware in working with Jennifer that I was fundamentally dealing with a developing identity and not a psychiatric condition, long before there was a legal recognition of these new identities in many countries. A question remains: what conferred continuity to his atypical gender identity development?

This case shows that the combination of an exploratory and accepting attitude, could be a good approach in terms of promoting well-being. In this case the main focus of the work was the amelioration of the associated psychosocial difficulties. I later realized that these are present in a number of cases. Reflection on this case led to the original formulation of the therapeutic aims in work with children with gender diversity and their families (Di Ceglie, 1998).

The therapeutic aims were summarized as follows:

(1) *To foster recognition and non-judgemental acceptance of gender identity issues.*
(2) *To ameliorate associated behavioural, emotional and relationship difficulties.*
(3) *To break the cycle of secrecy.*
(4) *To activate interest and curiosity by exploring the impediments to them.*
(5) *To encourage exploration of the mind-body relationship by promoting close collaboration among professionals in different specialities, including paediatric endocrinology.*
(6) *To allow mourning processes to occur.*
(7) *To enable symbol formation and symbolic thinking.*
(8) *To promote separation and differentiation.*
(9) *To enable the child or adolescent and the family to tolerate uncertainty in gender identity development.*
(10) *To sustain hope.*

It is important to add to this list the need to combat stigma which is often associated with the experience of atypical gender identity and which is, at times, internalized by the individual experiencing GD.

It is also valuable to alleviate the feeling of shame that some children/adolescents and their family experience and enable people to develop skills in handling social interaction and dealing with possible hostility.

This therapeutic approach is developmentally based, is not prescriptive, addresses the young person's distress and aims at promoting well-being. It is not part of reparative/conversion therapy and has elements of affirmative therapy.

In one of the last sessions after two years of exploratory therapy, Jennifer said that perhaps this form of help had come too late and that her parents should have been aware of how she was feeling by the way she behaved as a child. She wondered why they had not sought help at that time. Jennifer's thoughts made me wonder why there was no service for children with these rare, unusual and distressing experiences. This planted in me the seed for the creation of such a service. About three years after, GIDS was established in the department of child psychiatry in 1989 at St Georges Hospital in South London. In 1996, the service transferred to the Tavistock and Portman Trust (Di Ceglie, 2021).

Case 2

Britton (1998), in his book *Belief and Imagination*, distinguishes between beliefs and fantasies. He states: 'Beliefs have consequences: they arouse feelings, influence perception and promote actions ... Fantasies, conscious or unconscious, which are not the object of belief, do not have consequences: disavowal therefore can be used to evade these consequences' (Britton, 1998, p. 11).

Therapeutic exploration will help to clarify these two different states of mind. The following interaction illustrates the level of conviction of belief of a 13-year-old, assigned female at birth whose self-perception was of being a boy. This interaction occurred in a family session involving the mother, the step-father, the young person called Max, a child psychotherapist colleague and myself. The session was recorded for a documentary in 1994.

The metaphor, which I use in the following clip, came to my mind after reading an article by Jan Morris 'On the sadness of living abroad'. Here Morris describes the psychological experience of some English people who had migrated to France. Today we could call this experience 'the migrant dysphoria'. She says:

> It is not just that I am sorry for the French, who are going to have to suffer the proximity of these cuckoos in the nest of the world; in a way I am sorrier for the English, who are going to turn themselves into expatriates. All over the world one sees them, the islanders, evading their heritage, looking for the London newspapers in the Spanish newsagent, talking about duchesses at the New England Tennis Clubs, and, above all, almost anywhere beautiful in France, visiting each other's houses, remembering old times, comparing Major with Thatcher, Gooch with Botham. How happy they always say they are! How sad they generally seem to me. (Morris, 1991)

The following section is the transcript of a clip from the documentary.

Female Therapist (FT): What would you like to be called?
Max: Now? It's certainly not Sarah.
FT: What would you like us to call you?
Max: I don't know.
Mother (M): We just call Max, Max. But when I hear somebody else calling her, Sarah, or something, I just . . .
Max: Why do you say 'her'?
M: Sorry, sorry.
Father: That's the hardest bit . . .
M: It's the 'he' and the 'she' because it's really difficult and I feel weird calling Max 'her' or 'she'. Yeah. (To Max) I feel weird calling you it.
FT: Is that the bit that hurts the most?
Max: Yes. (M) says it all the time.
M: I do. I do. Yeah.
FT: But do you feel (hurt) with your mother or with everyone?
Max: No, [Male Therapist] calls me it too.
FT: Does it hurt the same?
Max: Yes.
FT: It hurts the same.
Max: Yes.
M: I know you'd rather be called 'he' but I do try, promise, we both do.
Male Therapist (MT): But I think it is a difficult issue to tackle because it's a bit similar to an English boy, born in England, brought up in England, about 15, 16, who emigrates to France and then goes around and says to everybody that I'm French. That I want to be considered French. While his accent will show that he is not French. So this is . . .
Max: No, that's not it though, because he wants to be, he isn't, but I am.
MT: But that is one of the problems because, of course, what your body says is different from what you feel inside you are. Like in this person, what he would like to be is French and this is different from what his accent, at least, you know, no other features . . .
Max: I don't want to be, I don't like to be . . . a boy.
FT: You are a boy?
Max: Yes.

An extract from another session shows further the strength of the conviction of this teenager and the difficulties in tolerating uncertainty or that the mother could have another point of view.

M: Max has asked us specifically on several occasions not to call him Sarah because we have called him Max since he was incy, and to say 'he' and not 'she'. And he's explained that it really, really hurts when someone says 'she'. And also it's ever so complicated if I introduce him as 'she' because people think I've gone mad so ...
Max: You sound as if you're just doing it ...
M: Because you've asked me to ...
Max: Yeah, one of the reasons. Why aren't you doing it for you?
M: Also for me, because eventually if you do go ahead and have all the treatment I'm gonna have ...
Max: Why do you say 'if'?
M: Well, all right then, 'when'. I'm gonna look pretty stupid if I'm the only person on the planet calling you 'she'.
Max: You sound as if you're just worried about what you do.
M: No, it's for you and for everybody. What you need to understand is that it takes some time for somebody like me to readjust and I do try, really, really, hard because the last thing I want is to upset you ...
MT: The important point that you are making is that you feel that there should be no doubt about who you are ...
Max: Yeah.
MT: ... in this case you feel that you are a boy and there should be no doubt that you are a boy. And when you pick up any doubt about it, or that people are uncertain about it, that's very upsetting for you ...

Max's perception of his male gender identity persisted until he was in contact with the service. At 18 he pursued further treatment in an adult service.

This case shows the value of a psychotherapeutic exploration in helping to distinguish between gender identity presentations which are more solid and presentations which are more fluid and changeable. The material from this case in particular, enabled the formulation of the so-called 'atypical gender identity organization' (AGIO) (Di Ceglie, 1998).

The characteristics of the organization are as follows:

(a) *Rigidity–flexibility or solidity–fluidity of the AGIO. This refers to the capacity of the atypical gender identity organisation of the individual to remain unchangeable or, alternatively, along a continuum, to be amenable to evolution in the course of development. Organisations which are more rigid or solid will contribute to the persistence/continuity of the atypical gender identity development, while organisations which are more flexible or fluid will lead to shifts in gender identity development. In about 10–30% of pre-pubertal children the gender dysphoria persists into adolescence. After puberty, the persistence/continuity into adulthood is much higher.*

(b) *Timing of the AGIO formation. Atypical Gender Identity Organisations that develop very early in the child's life may be more likely to become solidly structured than organisations that develop later. The early onset of gender dysphoria is in fact one of the criteria for considering early pubertal suppression.*

(c) *Traumatic events in childhood. It can be hypothesized that in some cases an AGIO may be formed as a psychological coping strategy in relation to a traumatic event in childhood. The earlier the trauma occurs, the more likely it is that the organisation will acquire unchangeable qualities.*
(d) *Position on the paranoid-schizoid-depressive continuum. The Klein-Bion model of psychological development posits a continuum from the paranoid–schizoid to the depressive positions. An individual oscillates between these two positions or mental states. Precisely where the child's mental state resides along this continuum when an AGIO is formed is of significance. The hypothesis here is that if the AGIO is formed during a period of development within the mental functioning of the paranoid – schizoid position, it is more likely to become very structured, have the quality of a solid identity and therefore be less amenable to change. Alternatively, if it is formed within a mental functioning of the depressive position it is likely that the organisation will have more fluid qualities (fluid identity) and be amenable to evolution.*

Therapeutic exploration may be able to elucidate the characteristics of the organization or the shape of gender identity of that particular individual and therefore guide management.

Case 3

Martin was referred in the early 1990s to the Gender Identity Development Service (GIDS) at the age of eight when he was attending a primary school. The educational psychologist reported that his mother said that he had told her when he was seven that he wanted to be a woman when he grew up. He enjoyed dressing in women's clothing and, ever since he could walk, he liked to wear high heels and use tea towels to mimic long hair. He was very fond of Barbie dolls and his mannerisms and style of walking were feminine. At school he played only with girls. He lacked confidence and was teased by other children, who called him offensive names. He suffered from symptoms of anxiety including stomach upsets, dizziness and headaches. His mother did not encourage his feminine behaviour but was supportive.

During his assessment at GIDS, we confirmed that Martin presented the features of a well-established gender identity disorder (now gender dysphoria in DSM-5). His anxiety about attending school resulted in poor attendance, and he also experienced teasing on the estate where he lived. He also had difficulties separating from his mother. At our service, we started working closely with the family, which consisted of Martin, his mother and his stepfather and had meetings with the school staff to facilitate his attendance at school.

Two years later Martin moved with his family to another town in England. Here, his wish to live in a female role became very intense and the parents agreed to let him live as a girl, expressed by dressing in female clothes and changing his name to Martina.

In her new town, Martina became involved in individual therapeutic work with a community nurse in the local child and adolescent mental health service (CAMHS). A colleague and I continued to see the parents every two months to help them to reflect on the gender identity and other developmental issues involved and to be able to make more informed decisions with their child (parental counselling). The parents attended a group for parents of GD children for six months (Di Ceglie & Coates Thümmel, 2006). We continued to hold regular professional network meetings, including the school staff, two or three times a year. Martina attended a small special educational unit in a female role, following careful preparation and discussions of the issues involved between the professional network (including us) and the family.

When Martina was 13, the Social Services Department called a child protection conference as the school had become concerned that parental attitudes could have contributed to the development of Martina's gender dysphoria. After an investigation and a child protection conference, no child protection issues were found. As a result of this conference, the mother was offered further supportive individual counselling by local services.

When Martina was 14, while waiting to be seen by our paediatric endocrinologist, as she was entering puberty, she unexpectedly announced to her mother that she no longer wished to be a girl, and she now felt happier about being a boy. From then on, Martina reverted to living as Martin. The next time I saw him he had physically developed a lot and had the clear appearance of a boy. At the last professional/family network meeting I asked Martin if he thought that his parents had made a wrong decision in allowing him to attend school in a female role and he replied without hesitation that it had been right because that was how he had felt at the time (DiCeglie, 2018b).

From this case, which I saw in the 1990s, I drew the following conclusion:

(1) *Pubertal development can sometimes, even in well-established cases of gender dysphoria, change the course of gender identity development.*
(2) *A parental response, which goes along with the intense wishes of the child to live in the perceived gender identity and role, does not necessarily influence the course of gender identity development. However, maintaining an open mind facilitates the process of change if this occurs.*
(3) *My professional role was to maintain a reflective approach in working with the family and the professional network, evaluating pros and cons,*

> *and to facilitate decision- making within the family regarding what was in the best interests of the child in that particular social context.*

There is very limited research evidence to suggest which approach to children living in their preferred gender role (social transition) during childhood is best. Long-term follow-up studies have shown that only in a small proportion (up to 30%) of pre-pubertal children presenting with the features of gender dysphoria, did the gender dysphoria continue through adolescence and adulthood with or without any therapeutic intervention (Cohen-Kettenis, 2001; Green et al., 1987; Zucker & Bradley, 1995; Drummond et al., 2008; Wallien & Cohen-Kettenis, 2008). Steensma et al. (2011, p. 1) suggest that among young people who changed: 'the period between 10 and 13 years of age was considered to be crucial ... Both persisters and desisters stated that the changes in their social environment, the anticipated and actual feminization or masculinization of their bodies, and their first experiences of falling in love and sexual attraction, had influenced their gender related interest, behaviour, feelings of gender discomfort, and gender identification'.

My initial thinking about the management of gender role and social transition in childhood were based on a long-term observation of the case described from the 1990s. Since then, I have seen a number of pre-pubertal children and found that the exercise of autonomy in decision-making on the part of the parents and the child has been a helpful policy. The provision of a therapeutic exploration, jointly with the family and a neutral professional, is helpful. The exploration would aim at enhancing the capacity for autonomy in the family and, in this way, lead to better informed consent to what is in the best interests for the development of the child and in particular of their gender identity. The value of therapeutic explorations and counselling with young people and their families could be seen from a new vertex: 'their role in the service of the ethical principle of autonomy and better-informed decision-making'. Long-term follow-ups and further research in this area can contribute to the continuous development of appropriate guidelines.

Conclusion

In this paper I have tried to show how reflecting over a period of time on case material, as Bonnard did with painting, can allow a process of 'learning from experience' in the words of Bion and contribute to the development of models of care for different shapes of atypical gender identity. As clinical experiences and research evidence evolve, so will models of care.

The management of gender dysphoria in a number of young people may require for the young person and the family decision making regarding hormonal intervention. There is a risk, in our digital age and current cultural climate, that the process of evaluation and assessment becomes rather mechanical and simplistic. The role of

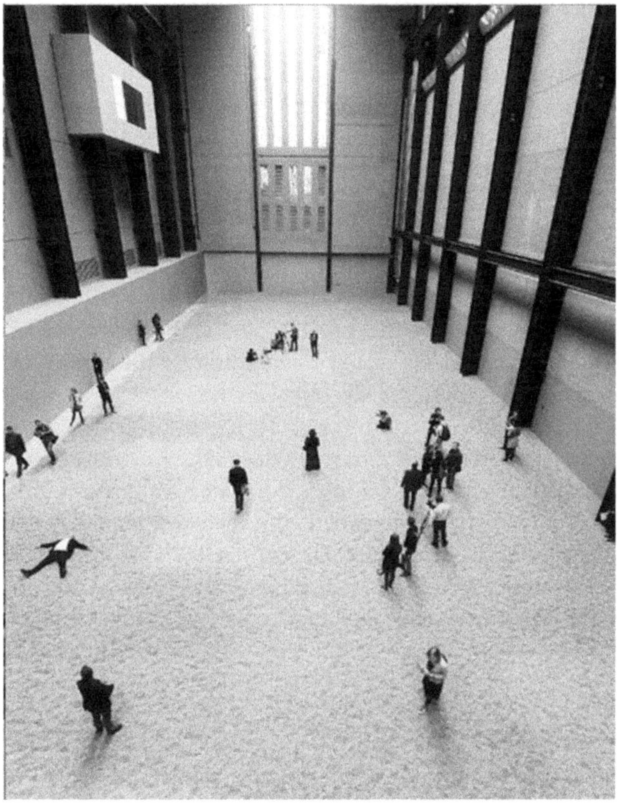

Figure 2. At a distance: an apparent undifferentiated mass of sunflower seeds.

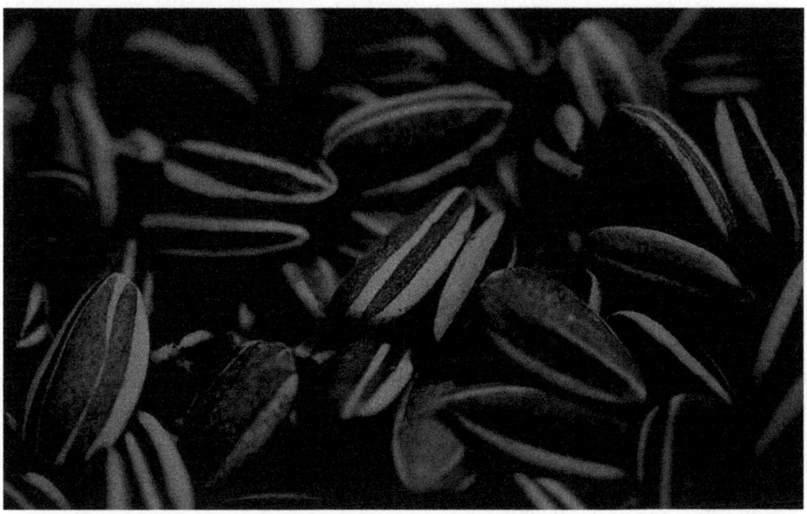

Figure 3. Close up: the uniqueness of each individual seed.

therapeutic exploration may be to promote the development of autonomy and better-informed decision making in young people and their families.

I would like to end with a metaphor which stimulates a reflection on the nature of gender diversity in children. Recently, the Chinese artist Ai Weiwei created an installation at the Tate Modern in London which he called *Sunflower Seeds*.

This extensive mass of seeds (120 million) seen at a distance looks uniform and undifferentiated (see Figure 2), but as one looks a bit more closely, the individuality of each seed becomes more and more evident (see Figure 3).

There are no two seeds which are the same.

Ai Weiwei explained that each porcelain seed was individually painted by workers, who collaborated in the project, and not by a machine. Each seed required between three and six strokes according to the ability or the style of each collaborator. Therefore, the diversity of the seeds was the result of the creative process (DiCeglie, 2018a).

In a way similar to this work of art, children who present with atypical gender identity development, ('gender dysphoria', in DSM-5) all present differently within this category and not as part of a stereotype. It is therefore important to offer different types of help according to a range of diverse needs. 'One size fits all' cannot be applied to this group, instead, as professionals and society, we should respond empathically and flexibly to the particular experiences and story of each young person.

Disclosure statement

No potential conflict of interest was reported by the author(s).

Disclaimer

Every effort has been made to identify and contact the copyright holders for the use of copyright material. The author/publisher would be pleased to rectify any omissions in future editions should they be drawn to our attention.

References

Britton, R. (1998). *Belief and imagination*. Routledge.

Cohen-Kettenis, P.T. (2001). Gender Identity Disorder in DSM? *Journal of the American Academy of Child and Adolescent Psychiatry, 40*(4), 391.

Di Ceglie, D. (1998). Management and therapeutic aims with children and adolescents with gender identity disorders and their families. In D. Di Ceglie, and D. Freedman (Eds.), *A stranger in my own body: Atypical gender identity development and mental health* (pp. 185-197). Karnac Books.

Di Ceglie, D. (2018a). The use of metaphors in understanding atypical gender identity development and psychosocial impact. *Journal of Child Psychotherapy, 44*(1), 5–28. https://doi.org/10.1080/0075417X.2018.1443151

Di Ceglie, D. (2018b). Autonomy and decision-making in children and adolescents with gender dysphoria. In M. Shaw, and S. Bailey (Eds.), *Justice for children and families – A developmental perspective* (p. 151). Cambridge University Press.

Di Ceglie, D. (2021). The creation of a service for children and adolescents facing gender identity issues. In M. Waddell & S. Kraemer (Eds.), *The Tavistock Century: 2020 Vision* (pp. 159–164). Phoenix.

Di Ceglie, D., & Coates Thümmel, E. (2006). An experience of groupwork with parents of children and adolescents with gender identity disorder. *Clinical Child Psychology and Psychiatry, 11*(3), 387–396. https://doi.org/10.1177/1359104506064983

Di Ceglie, D., Skagerberg, E., Baron-Cohen, S., & Auyeung, B. (2014). Emphathising and systemising in adolescents with gender dysphoria. *Opticon 1826*, *16*(6), 1–8. https://doi.org/10.5334/opt.bo

Drummond, K. D., Bradley, S. J., Peterson-Badali, M., & Zucker, K. J. (2008). A follow up study of girls with gender identity disorder. *Developmental Psychology*, *44*(1), 34–45. https://doi.org/10.1037/0012-1649.44.1.34

Gale, M. (2019). *Pierre Bonnard – The colour of memory*. The CC Land Exhibition, Exhibition guide, Tate Modern, 23 January-6 May 2019.

Green, R., Roberts, C.W., Williams, R., Goodman , M., and Mixon, A. (1987). Specific cross-gender behaviour in boyhood and later homosexual orientation. *British Journal of Psychiatry*, *151*, 84–88.

Jones, R., Wheeelwright, S., Farrell, K., Martin, E., Green, R., Di Ceglie, D., & Baron-Cohen, S. (2012). Female-to-male transsexual people and autistic traits. *Journal of Autism and Developmental Disoders*, *42*(2), 301–306. https://doi.org/10.1007/s10803-011-1227-8

Morris, J. (1991, October 19). On the sadness of living abroad. *The Independent Magazine*.

Skagerberg, E., Di Ceglie, D., & Carmichael, P. (2015). Brief report: Autistic features in children and adolescents with gender dysphoria. *Journal of Autism and Developmental Disorders*, *45*(8), 2628–2632. https://doi.org/10.1007/s10803-015-2413-x

Steensma, T. D., Biemond, R., De Boer, F., & Cohen-Kettenis, P. T. (2011). Desisting and persisting gender dysphoria after childhood: A qualitative follow up study. *Clinical Child Psychology and Psychiatry*, *16*(4), 499–516. https://doi.org/10.1177/1359104510378303

Wallien, M. S. C., & Cohen-Kettenis, P. T. (2008). Psychosexual outcome of gender dysphoric children. *Journal of the American Academy of Child and Adolescent Psychiatry*, *47*(12), 1413–1423. https://doi.org/10.1097/CHI.0b013e31818956b9

Zucker, K., & Bradley, S. J. (1995). *Gender identity disorder and psychosexual problems in children and adolescents*. Guildford Press.

Between partnering and parenting: psychoanalytic approaches to working with parental couples

Andrew Balfour

This paper explores the link between parenting difficulties and couple relationship issues in psychotherapeutic work with parental couples. Initially, the discussion focusses on the social policy context of couple psychotherapy and the resistances it can evoke, which has led to an emphasis on 'parenting' rather than 'couple' interventions in the historic development of family service provision in the UK. Some developmental challenges facing couples who are parents are then discussed, focussing on a clinical case and drawing on the concepts of shared unconscious phantasy and enactment in the analytic session, to elucidate defensive and developmental possibilities of working at the interface between 'parenting' and 'partnering'.

The organisational setting: Tavistock Relationships

The work described in this paper took place at Tavistock Relationships, an organisation providing couple psychotherapy and practitioner training whose approach is rooted in psychoanalysis. In the 100 years since the birth of the Tavistock Clinic, a number of organisations have been part of the wider 'Tavistock family' of institutions. These have included: Tavistock Institute of Human Relations, the Tavistock Institute of Medical Psychology, the Tavistock Career and Education Consultation Service, as well as Tavistock Relationships which was founded in 1948 as the Family Discussion Bureau by social workers from the Family Welfare Association and psychoanalysts at The Tavistock Clinic who shared an ambition to study the dynamics of family life. Tavistock Relationships' parent body, the Tavistock Institute of Medical Psychology, is the founding organisation that set up the Tavistock Clinic in 1920. Throughout its lifetime, Tavistock Relationships has been a 'sister' organisation to the Clinic, with a history of personal and professional links and sharing a common approach of rigorous grounding in clinical work as a basis for research, training and the application of analytic thinking to the broadest range of human problems; a mission to reach people and touch areas of human experience that have not before had the benefit of analytic understanding. It is this distinctive 'Tavistock approach', with its focus on developmental challenges and developmental possibilities throughout the lifespan, which has been at the heart of the work of Tavistock Relationships since its inception.

The social policy context

Couples often come for help around the time of becoming parents, perhaps unconsciously perceiving the psychic challenges the arrival of a child will bring; often, expressing the poignant wish that they will not pass on the problems they had in their own families, when they were growing up, to their children. They are not wrong in recognising the importance of this, as research shows us that the quality of the parental couple's relationship, in particular whether this is characterised by intense and unresolved conflict, is crucial in shaping children's outcomes – their health, well-being and long-term development (Harold & Leve, 2012). For many years, this was held to be only an indirect effect, consequent on the impact of couples' relationship difficulties on their parenting capacity. Now, however, the research evidence confirms what, psychoanalytically, we always knew: there is a direct impact of exposure to parental relationship problems upon children, as the external atmosphere of the family becomes internalized as part of the inner lived world of the child, often then reproduced in their relationships with others. Indeed, there is now a convergence of evidence, from developmental and social research as well as from our consulting rooms, which shows us that the parental couple relationship is the crucible of our mental health – for children, as well as for the adults themselves (see A. Balfour et al., 2012).

When parental couples do seek help, how do our services respond to them? Often, rather than being offered couple psychotherapy, they will be referred to a 'parenting programme'. Parenting work has been more acceptable, and much more commonly available, than couple psychotherapy in most British settings. Within our NHS Child and Family Services, it is the only intervention that is routinely available to parental couples, even though parenting programmes do not directly address the parents' relationship difficulties, and we know how counter-productive it can be to undertake parenting work with a couple who are in significant conflict, without attending to the couple relationship issues themselves (Harold & Leve, 2012). Indeed, family relationship problems were amongst the most frequently cited issues by children of all age groups who contacted a leading charity, 'Childline' (Komaromi, 2019), and a survey of Children's Mental Health Services undertaken by Tavistock Relationships (Meier, 2018), indicated that parental couple difficulties were a significant underlying factor in over half of all the cases they were seeing. Resistance to allowing a couple focus into health and social care settings means that our human services tend to have an 'atomized' focus, on the individual in isolation, with 'siloed' working evident in the chasm that exists between the worlds of adult and children's mental health. And yet, the couple relationship is at the heart of the family, and this has been recognised in the work of Tavistock Relationships since its beginning as the Family Discussion Bureau at the end of WW2, at a time when the social disruption of war had wreaked profound problems on families across the world.

In the UK, government funders are now becoming more convinced by the research evidence which shows the impact of inter-parental conflict on children's long term development, as well as the effectiveness of couple-focussed psychotherapy. For example, longitudinal research shows that the quality of the couple relationship is a crucial indicator of how well the couple will function as parents, and also highlights the superior, beneficial effect of couple intervention compared to only parenting focussed work, in improving both couple and child outcomes (Cowan & Pape Cowan, 2009). The building research evidence base is now shifting the position of couple psychotherapy within the mental health field. We can now unequivocally state that entrenched and unresolved inter-parental conflict is profoundly damaging for children's development (Harold et al., 2001; Meier, 2018), and we can also demonstrate that we can intervene effectively to improve the situation (Hewison et al., 2016). And yet, despite this research evidence, interventions that seek to help the couple relationship are still the poor relation to those directly targeting parenting skills. Why should this be? Anxieties about intervening with the adult couple often run very deep; it can be a daunting business, facing the clinician with complex feelings, to do with our own experiences of couple relationships, and of negotiating the original parental relationship of our earliest years. At Tavistock Relationships we often receive referrals from social workers and others engaged in parenting work who feel out of their depth if issues to do with the couple's relationship threaten to come into the therapy. This reluctance to attend to the couple relationship can be found at all levels: from the individual worker, to commissioners, policy makers, and couples themselves.

Indeed, problems with children, or parenting issues, can often be the 'ticket' for couples' entry into therapeutic services. Sometimes, in our projects, when trying to encourage people who hitherto may not have had access to relationship support, we have found it is more acceptable to offer 'parental couple' help, rather than 'couple therapy'. For example, we called our service for parents experiencing high levels of conflict in their couple relationship 'Parenting under Pressure'. And of course, where there are family problems children can often be the ones who act as 'lightning conductors' for this, whose behaviour may be unconsciously intended to draw attention to the family's need for help. The manifest problem may then be felt as residing in one of the children who are acting out in such a way, with the parental couple problems underpinning the wider systemic difficulties in the family. Offering services for couples with a focus on their role as parents can sometimes make it easier for them to come for help and it can then become acceptable – over time – for them to allow the focus to shift to their relationship. Nevertheless, within the clinical work, it can be a delicate balance, moving from real and important parenting concerns, to an engagement in troubled couple dynamics – which themselves interact with, which shape and are shaped by, children's problems. I shall shortly discuss a clinical case to illustrate this, but first, let us think about some of the developmental challenges that face couples in being parents.

Developmental challenges of being parents

As I have said, couples often become parents hoping to do things differently in their new family and not to pass on intergenerational difficulties to their own children. Yet, as a consequence of the challenges of parenthood, they may find themselves repeating some version of the past, even in their very efforts to avoid it. Although, of course, becoming parents for the first time is to journey into a new world, the couple are faced with something that, in a sense, is not new. Becoming parents faces all couples with fundamental developmental challenges, of moving from two to three. The Oedipus situation, of a parental couple and a child, has lived inside them, in various guises at different developmental points, throughout their lives. As they step across the generational divide to become parents themselves, it is now realised in a new form. How this developmental challenge is negotiated will depend upon the internal legacy of earlier times, and on the extent to which the original Oedipus situation of infancy has been worked through.

Writing more than 100 years ago, in his novel, *The Rainbow*, DH Lawrence describes a young child's reaction to her mother's relationship with her new husband, now the child, Anna's, stepfather. Whilst the situation of a mother's new relationship may bring particular challenges, this description evokes the painful difficulty of the Oedipus situation that we all know from our personal experience:

> Anna wriggled close into her mother's arms, clinging tight, hiding from the fact of the man … "Go away," came the sharp little command … .
> "You can't send your father from his own bed, my little bird," said her mother, pleasantly.
> The child glowered at him, miserable in her impotence.
> "There's room for you as well," he said. "It's a big bed, enough."
> She glowered without answering, then turned and clung to her mother. She would not allow it … "Why do you sleep with my mother? My mother sleeps with me," her voice quivering.
> Her mother said: " … I must have a husband, darling. All women must have a husband"
> "And you like to have a father with your mother, don't you?" (he) said.
> Anna glowered at him. She seemed to cogitate.
> "No," she cried fiercely at length, "no, I don't want."
> (D.H. Lawrence, *The Rainbow*, pp. 64-65)

The 'Oedipus Complex' is one of the best known, but, perhaps in the popular imagination, least understood psychoanalytic concepts. It has entered into the vernacular, associated with themes of mother-love, sex and rivalry. However, Freud's account was central to the development of his theory of mind; the beginning of an account of the processes of internalization and introjection and the development of different agencies within the mind, particularly the ego ideal, which later became an aspect of the superego. Klein's work developed our understanding of what she termed the 'Oedipus Situation' (Klein 1928), in which she included the sexual relation between the parents, which Freud had considered in the context of the 'primal scene'. She positioned the developmental conflict inherent in the Oedipus Complex much earlier in life, as experienced by the infant at the oral and anal stages of development as well as at the genital stage of Freud's original formulation. In doing so, Klein re-visioned the Oedipus Situation as concerned with relations between objects as they are coloured by unconscious phantasy (a term which I shall explain below), moving away from the classical emphasis on the distribution of psychic energies, towards a theory of internal object relations. As I shall describe, her work has been developed by post-Kleinian thinkers in ways which have helped us to understand how early developmental difficulties in the Oedipus Situation can return to dominate the psychic life of the couple and, perhaps most of all, this can be evident as they become parents themselves.

How is it that early difficulties in negotiating the Oedipus situation lead to problems for the couple who are becoming parents? Although, of course, it is never, for any of us 'resolved' in any final sense, working through the Oedipus situation under optimal conditions entails, as Britton (1989, p. 86) puts it: '*The acknowledgement by the child of the parents' relationship with each other (which) unites his psychic world*'; establishing, that is, the ability to know about a relationship that one is linked to, but which exists separately to the self. Britton (1989, p. 87) writes: 'If the link between the parents ... can be tolerated in the child's mind, it provides him with a prototype for an object relationship of a third kind in which he is a witness and not a participant. A third position then comes into existence from which object relationships can be observed. Given this, we can also envisage being observed.' The idea here is that this developmental achievement brings the emotional maturity to establish a 'linked separateness' to the object, the ability to be able to inhabit a relationship and also to move, psychically, to a vantage point from which one can observe this relationship and one's place within it. This describes the capacity to be both *in* the relationship, but also *outside* and so able to reflect upon it, establishing what is termed a 'third position' in relation to the object. This is a significant developmental shift, enabling the emotional flexibility to view one's relationships from different perspectives, to be able to make mental movements within 'triangular' psychic space. Without this developmental achievement, the couple may inhabit a more 'binary' psychic space, where they find it difficult to establish an intimacy in which each partner can feel securely connected with one another, but also anchored in their own separate identities. Unable to establish the 'linked separateness' which Britton describes, they may struggle to regulate emotional distance and psychic space between them, tending either to feel 'too close', or 'too far away' from one another, fearful of being suffocated and 'swallowed up' or else left out and abandoned (Balfour, 2005; Rey, 1994). Psychoanalytic accounts of such 'claustro-agoraphobic' anxieties (see Birkstead-Breen, 1996; Britton, 1989; Glasser, 1979) describe how these may be the consequence of early difficulties in the dyadic link of infant with mother, which amplify for the child the challenges of tolerating the Oedipal link between the parents, and compound the problems of working through the Oedipus situation. These writers outline how the developmental legacy of this may be the anxiety that psychic intercourse, the bringing together of two psychic realities in an intimate relationship, will be catastrophic.

For the adult couple, then, difficulties in this area of development are linked to fears about intimate relating. Commonly, for a couple who inhabit such a 'binary world' the leading anxiety may be that the bringing together of two minds in 'psychic intercourse' threatens the obliteration of one by the other, and their experience is that there is room only for one point of view, one mind, within their relationship. Arguments can have a 'life or death' quality, as they fight over whose will dominate, which partner's version of experience will be accepted as the 'Truth'. As the therapist, you may feel that if you try to understand one partner you are ignoring, or even negating, the other. Within the session, there is an absence of psychic space and it is very hard to find any vantage point from which to observe and reflect. Needless to say, this situation is very different from working with a couple who have achieved a more mature working through of the Oedipus situation which, as Britton describes, enables the capacity to reflect on their own experience and that of their partner, as well as on the relationship between them. In the clinical setting with a couple where such psychic development has been achieved, there is the freedom to make mental movements between different vantage points, an experience of 'psychic space' in the session, which allows each partner's experience to be taken in and reflected upon without causing existential threat to self or other.

What is the significance of difficulties in this area of development for a couple who are becoming parents? Problems in negotiating the original Oedipus situation will make a difficult business of entering into the triangular situation of becoming a parental couple, which means that their relationship will struggle to function as a creative container for the adult partners, and for the baby who enters into this relationship with them. The normal fluctuating inclusions and exclusions of adults and child in shifting permutations of coupling, of mother-baby, father-mother, father-baby, which are characteristic of family life, will be difficult to tolerate. As part of the legacy of such developmental difficulties, the couple may feel, at an unconscious level, that they cannot be both parents and a couple – that there cannot be a couple, with their own separate life, and a child. Couples with problems in this area may present as parents who are entirely focussed on their child and as though they themselves do not exist as a couple; or conversely, they may take up an exclusive preoccupation with their relationship, excluding the child. Whilst, on the face of it, these presenting issues look somewhat different they share a common underlying factor: the developmental difficulty of inhabiting a triangular relational situation, where the parents have their own relationship which is separate from, but linked to, the child. These psychoanalytic accounts help us to understand how, in working with couples who are struggling with such developmental difficulties and presenting with problems in being parents, the task is not only to understand their struggles in managing the threesome of parents and child, but also to think about how these link with the difficulty of being a twosome – the anxieties about coupling within the parental couple's relationship with one another. I shall try to bring these ideas to life now, showing how they help us to understand and work psychotherapeutically with couples.

Working with a couple

In the interests of confidentiality this case example is anonymised and draws on work with a number of couples whose experiences have been amalgamated. I have tried, nonetheless, to do this in a way which still gives the essence of an authentic experience of working with couples who have difficulties in this area of their development. Although I am describing couple psychoanalytic work with a 'nuclear family', I believe that these ideas have a much wider relevance to other settings and configurations of relationships. Readers of this article may be working in various settings and I think parents may be helped if those who are working with them have these ideas in mind in contexts which may be very different from that of formal psychotherapy. In our work, we might be alert to oedipal configurations at different developmental stages. For example, when the first baby arrives claustrophobic aspects can be part of maternal post-natal depression. Father may feel on the outside and withdraw in response to this experience, leaving mother and baby in a more claustrophobic position. And, at different stages of development there might be a variety of configurations on this theme. I hope that this case example will help to bring these concepts to life for the reader and enable you to think about how they might be 'translated' into work which is taking place in other settings.

I shall focus on exploring the relationship between presenting parental concerns and underlying couple problems in the discussion of psychotherapeutic work with a young couple. Their presenting issues around parenting were, I came to feel, underlain by problems in establishing the capacity for 'triangular psychic space', linked to difficulties within the dyadic relationship of the couple which underpinned their problems in being partners as well as becoming parents.

Not parents and partners: the emergence of an unconscious belief

Barbara and Anthony were a young professional couple. They were seen for weekly psychotherapy at Tavistock Relationships, which offers a psychoanalytic psychotherapy clinic for couples. Coming for psychotherapy was, for them, a very difficult step to take. Their presenting problems focussed on their son, aged twelve, and caused them considerable shame and embarrassment; they should, as professionals, be able to sort things out, they felt, and this was linked to powerful feelings of guilt which further disabled their functioning as parents. All of their early sessions focussed on their son and his problems and it felt that to exclude him as the focus of preoccupation would be catastrophic in some way. At this stage, it seemed that the only version of a couple that was allowed was an anxious, worried parental couple. In this period, they presented as living parallel lives, focussed on their child and their anxieties made it very difficult for them to hold onto the sense of themselves as a couple, that they couldn't be partners as well as parents. It seemed that their reparative efforts, to ensure that he did not have the depriving experience that they had had themselves as children, meant that they had to sacrifice their own needs, and in so doing, maintained the sense of deprivation that they had felt all of their lives.

On one occasion, when at last, they were on a rare evening out together, their son phoned them and said would they come back, because he was feeling bad and needed them. When I queried this, they both said, with some pride, that they didn't hesitate but offer to come back. It seemed there was no thought that they might be able to help him, and also hold onto their evening together – they had to give up what they had, as a couple, and put their child at the centre. We should be grateful, we are so lucky to have a child, they said. This mirrored the experience that they shared growing up as children themselves, of being subordinated to their parents' needs, and reproduced now the experience of supplying the needs of others, but neglecting their own. I felt that I could see how this expressed what Morgan (2017) has termed a shared unconscious belief – that there could be no parental need put ahead of a child's, that one set of needs could only be met at the cost of the other's. This was felt as an unquestionable reality, putting the child first and abnegating their own needs was something that any good parents would do, they asserted vehemently; it was not a belief that was open to being questioned or thought about. Although both went along with this, at times the resentment about it was felt within the couple relationship, where he would express his frustration at having to give up on things he wanted, and she would resent his doing so – she resenting his resentment, so to speak. Together, it seemed, they enacted a conflict between the competing needs of parent and child, so that what might have been a conflict internal to each of them, as to how to compromise between conflicting sets of needs that any parent must negotiate, became instead a polarised and static fight; one which expressed the phantasy of a 'zero-sum', where one person's needs could only be met at the cost of another's. In the stasis of the battle between them, they expressed the phantasy that any change in this situation would be a calamity – abdicating in this, any thinking about their anxieties about their own psychic development as individuals and as a couple.

In this account so far, I have referred to the couple's shared unconscious belief. Before going on to describe more of the work with Barbara and Anthony, I will outline what is meant by this and the related concept, of shared unconscious phantasy, as these are important ideas in understanding the clinical approach of couple psychoanalytic psychotherapy.

Shared unconscious phantasy and belief

In working with couples, we have the idea of *shared* unconscious phantasy. Within psychoanalysis, the concept of unconscious phantasy has developed as a way of understanding how, from the start of our lives, our inner worlds are built up by encoding phantasies of relationships between objects which populate our minds, and which are constantly worked and re-worked through cycles of projective and introjective identification. But what does it mean to say that unconscious phantasy is shared?

In falling in love, which some couples describe as the experience of 'meeting their soulmate', the couple may be unconsciously recognising the shared objects in their separate minds, apprehending at an unconscious level a commonality of inner experience which is linked to convergences between the unconscious phantasies held by each partner. These unconscious phantasies are not 'shared' in the sense of being the same, but rather, they have enough in common for us to say that they are 'shared' (see F. Balfour et al., 1986). Shared unconscious phantasy may be thought of as the 'glue' between a couple – the source of the unconscious attraction between partners on one hand, but on the other, the shared nature of this system can be a part of the problem. Shared areas of vulnerability and therefore shared anxieties, mean that the defences of each partner, which are often contrasting but complementary responses to shared underlying phantasies, can trigger one another and so become amplified. When this happens, the shared area of difficulty or vulnerability is more likely to become enacted between the partners. At times, one sees how the couple's defences fit together and enact key elements of their shared unconscious phantasy. Within the clinical setting, this may feel to the therapist rather like witnessing a repeated dramatization played out between the partners in a way which encapsulates and represents their shared fears and anxieties about intimate relationships. We might imagine the couple's 'stories' which they describe and live out within their sessions, as expressions of their shared unconscious phantasies about the nature of the dangers of intimate relating.

Where unconscious phantasies are inhabited in a way which is more fixed and less fluid and there is an absence of flexible identifying and dis-identifying with internal objects, this leads to a mode of functioning where unconscious phantasy will be experienced in a concrete way, having the quality of a belief that is an unchallengeable reality (Morgan, 2017). These more concretely held beliefs are less available for reflection and thought and so are more likely to be enacted by the couple. In the clinical setting, understanding enactment as it occurs within the couple and with the therapist, may be one way to get hold of shared unconscious phantasy and belief, if there is a convincing experience that crystallizes what the shared unconscious phantasy or belief is within the session. In this situation, the clinician is asking, what is it that is shared about their inner worlds that leads the couple to play out their internal conflicts and drama in this way? As I shall now try to show in my account of the next phase of the work with this couple, it is the emotional atmosphere within the clinical setting, the transference and counter-transference pushes and pulls, as well as the content of the material, that help us to develop a picture of the unconscious phantasies which are shared by the partners in their coupling.

Working with the couple's shared unconscious phantasy

Returning now to Barbara and Anthony, at this stage in the work with them I started to see that the usual dynamic of their relationship was that she was 'in retreat', whilst he 'pressed in'. The settled pattern was that she was seen as the one who rejected intimacy, whereas he wanted it, knowing always that he could rely on her to reject him. This captures something of how a couples' defences can 'fit' in a complementary way: on the one hand looking very different – she as not needing intimacy, he pushing for it and so providing an illusory confirmation of the adage that 'opposites attract'. And yet, as I came to understand it, these apparently different positions expressed their mutually reinforcing ways of managing the same underlying psychic situation, linked to their shared phantasies about the dangers of intimacy, which they enacted within the sessions – playing out together the situation of a retreat from emotional contact in the face of an intrusive object. What I felt was now becoming apparent was that, underlying the manifest presentation of problems with the three-cornered Oedipus situation, of a couple and a child, were anxieties arising out of early developmental difficulties, which were felt between the parental couple; fears, in particular, of claustrophobic invasion and psychic annihilation of the self – which emerged as a shared belief about the threat that intimacy entailed.

As the work went on, whenever there was a move away from the parental focus, I found it was hard to get space to think within the session – and I could feel under pressure to line up with her or with him. I had difficulty in making interpretations to them based on my thoughts about what was happening, as though if I did so, I would wipe out one or other's experience. Sometimes, I would be felt to be doing just this – and the normally calm atmosphere would become explosive. I found myself treading warily in a situation where there was little psychic space, in a binary world where I was felt to be either 'with' him, or 'with' her. If I understood one partner's experience, I negated the other and there was only room for one mind, one point of view.

On one occasion, he spoke about his difficulty growing up in feeling he could have his own mind. His parents hadn't shown interest in things that he did, that were about him – only, in so far as those things fitted in with their own interests. This theme of feeling that there was no space for him in his family, for his mind, fitted with her experience – that had been explored recently – of how, whenever she was with her family of origin, she felt a kind of annihilation of her mind, of her thinking. Although there was a glimpse of something shared between them, at that moment in the room it felt more competitive than linked. At first, as he spoke, she made barbed comments – which I heard initially as dismissive, then as perhaps more prescient of the quality of what he was saying as he went on speaking: she said, she felt what he said wasn't real, somehow. Having initially felt critical of her for this, and protective of him, as he went on talking I started to agree with her in my mind, thinking he was 'fitting us in' to a narrative that had an emotionally absent quality. She was silent, letting him speak, apparently listening, but leaving the session to him. After a time, I took this up – how they both seemed to be behaving as if there was only space for one of them in the room. She said that she was aware of lots of feelings, but when he spoke she felt her own thoughts disappeared. She had nothing in her mind to say.

She seemed full of feelings – of difficult feelings, and most of all, that her thoughts were somehow annihilated as he was talking. She tried to engage, but, as she spoke, she would start and then stop. This was familiar, often she would halt at the moment she was about to get to the point – as if interrupted by an internal monitor – shut down just as she was about to express more meaningful thoughts or feelings. I took up the attacks that happened in her mind when she tried to speak, trying to put her head above the parapet, to allow her feelings to be seen. The retreat from emotional contact, which she expressed as a wiping out of her thoughts, which might be about to be tentatively voiced, but which were then negated, seemed to be part of a struggle in the room in which she was anguished and suffering.

By contrast, he appeared comfortable and composed, seeming to be in charge of himself and of his thoughts. As he went on speaking, I was aware of feeling invited into an apparently smooth and engaging narrative which then became drier and less engaging. I pointed out how comfortable he had seemed in telling us of his experience in a way which didn't seem to contain any of the feelings one might imagine he would have about it. At this point in the session, when I tried to put something of this into words, this produced a moment of acute anxiety in me – and, as I anticipated, he became very angry. He said that wasn't right at all – I had misunderstood him completely, and he went on at length explaining how wrong I had been. It felt that now, my attempts to reach him had to be rejected at all costs. His reaction had the quality of insistence and absolute certainty, his need to assert the 'correct' understanding, a life or death quality. I found it difficult to hold onto my thinking in the face of his response, momentarily losing a sense of anchorage in my perspective on what was happening between us in the room; perhaps given a taste of how it felt to have one's thoughts 'taken over'. Afterwards, in reflecting on what had happened, I felt that in this situation, where emotional contact with me, with my mind, seemed to be felt by him to threaten the annihilation of his, and where I felt that my own thinking was wiped out, we were in the territory of the shared unconscious phantasy. In my counter-transference, I had very direct experience of the phantasy that emotional contact threatened annihilation of mind. At this point in the session, whilst feeling provoked and realising that I was now enacting a coupling with him in which one mind, one psychic reality, had to dominate, I tried to think about this and to consider his complaints with him, and eventually this seemed to offer some containment in the heat of the session.

Whilst this was going on, she was quiet, observing the drama unfolding between him and me that she was used to encountering with him in their coupling. She commented: 'you and he are like him and me … it's exactly what it is like when he and I are fighting with one another. It's like looking in a mirror.' It seemed that she could find a vantage point from which to reflect on this familiar scenario as it was enacted without her at the centre of the action, as usually would be the case. She appeared to be thinking about what was happening in the session and then she came in with an association of her own. She spoke for the first time about her anxieties about sex, how she felt that she couldn't allow him to come near her, or to penetrate her – because it all seemed to be about him; she felt she didn't exist at all in those moments. She felt taken over, she said, as though he was trying to subsume her. I think this captured an image of the phantasy shared by them both – of the psychic takeover of one by another – that this was the expectation, and the threat, of what a relationship entailed. And it was this that I felt was often enacted between them and with me, as well as it was played out internally within each of them in the attacks on their minds, on allowing contact with a more open, vulnerable self, that I witnessed in the room with them.

In this example, when touching upon the area of unconscious phantasy, the quality of the session changed, and more absolute, unchallengeable 'certainties' about self and other emerged. The concreteness and absolute quality of the conviction that was expressed revealed this as an unconsciously held belief. When interpreting in this area, in ways which challenge the belief, and which therefore imply that there is more than one way of understanding or thinking about it, then the response is explosive. In this moment, the experience of such an interpretation in a sense enacts the very fear that is at the heart of the couple's unconscious phantasy or belief – an interpretation which is not only identified with the patient's experience, but is also an expression of links in the therapist's mind, with theory, clinical experience and an attempt to put these together to understand what is happening in relation to the couple. This attempt to reach the couple in a way that is connected to their experience, but also separate from it, can be felt to threaten to enact the very annihilation that they fear from such contact. This gives rise to very significant technical challenges, and one has to monitor the fate of interpretations and the response to them. Couples with difficulties in this area may not be functioning in a developmental position that would enable them to take in interpretations about what they are contributing to the dynamic between them, and with the therapist. Here, we need to consider the importance of what Steiner (1993) has termed 'analyst-centred' interpretations, which, in this context, we might think of as 'couple-experience centred' interpretations, which seek to understand the partners' experience of each other, and of the therapist and the therapy – whilst holding what Morgan (2001) terms a 'couple state of mind', so that they feel 'taken in' and understood, rather than being given interpretations that require them to take back in an understanding of themselves which they are not yet psychically equipped to do.

Efforts to offer an experience that I was open to his disturbing feelings and to thinking about his experience of me in the transference seemed to lead to a shift in the atmosphere in the room, with the emergence of confirmatory material. In observing what was happening between him and me, she seemed to find space to think, a 'third position' in relation to what was unfolding in the session, and her response at this point brought their shared unconscious phantasy more into the realm of thought. As time went on, the focus of the work shifted more to the dynamics of the couple relationship, and this development in the work faced me, as the therapist, with recognising my own part in having settled, for a time at least, for the 'quiet life' of restricting the field of vision to the worried parental couple, avoiding the significance of the 'not brought to life' sexual couple, and their deeper anxieties to do with their shared unconscious phantasies about the nature of intimate relating.

Development in the psychotherapeutic work with the couple

As these anxieties in the relationship between the parents began to be understood and worked through, the Oedipal couple came into view more clearly, expressed in unconscious phantasies which were initially emblematic of early, primitive versions of the Oedipus situation, conveyed in enactments and dream material within the sessions. For example, on one occasion, they told me about a row where he had felt overwhelmed with terrible feeling, unable to think, excluded and on the outside of the couple of his wife and son. They had gone out in the car, the three of them, with his feeling taken over by a sense of betrayal, of being on the outside of what he saw as their two-some, and, for a while, he had been unable to find a way back in. However, he said that, although he had been furious with her that evening, he had struggled in himself to think about it and had not been entirely taken over by these feelings. In the session, he thought about this and then added that he could see that, often, when she did try to get involved alongside him in parenting their son, he felt he had to intervene, to keep her out. He feared if she joined him in this it 'would make things worse' – things might go horribly wrong. I took this up, and was curious about what the catastrophe was that he feared. Their son might feel 'ganged up on, isolated and alone', he said. This was an image, not of parents coming together out of concern for their son, but one where the parental couple come together in a malign and excluding way. I pointed out to him that this was how he had felt – horribly excluded by his wife and son, feeling them to become such a couple – although he had also conveyed a capacity not to be taken over by his feelings, finding a way, eventually, to reflect on them.

Gradually, the difficulties of encompassing the triangular setting of the clinical situation and the familial one could be worked with, and more psychic separateness and life between the couple was able to emerge. On one occasion, she brought a dream. In this, she was with their son – though they were walking together and her son was a little apart from her. I was giving him some space and he looked different, she said, reflecting on this in the session. It was like I could see him from a different perspective; he looked more grown up. In the dream, she had then found herself in a building – a place where there were three large rooms, beside each other. She had gone and looked into them, and she had the thought that there was some life there, after all. She added, in the dream, it was like I could see my son differently – I was more separate. In this dream the three large rooms alongside each other are, perhaps, an image of the linked threesome of parents and child – a triangular situation that can now be brought together in the mind in a more benign, rather than paranoid, way; where the emotional atmosphere of the dream seems to be one of curiosity and excitement at the experience of a new vantage point, where a more separate psychic perspective is brought to life.

Alongside this, a clearer picture of their child came into the sessions, and I had a different perspective on him as I heard, not just about his difficulties, but also about his achievements – with parental pride, as well as concerns for his future, expressed in a more ordinary, realistic way . Only when this started to happen did I become aware of how absent their son had actually been in the sessions until this point, as he could now be seen as a more rounded, fully fleshed out person in his own right for the first time. I think this experience was reflective of the emergence of parents who were beginning to function as a creative couple together, more able to apprehend and take in the separate character and life of their son and to take pleasure in bringing this to life within our work together.

Conclusion

In summary, for much of the early period of work I had the feeling that Barbara and Anthony were missing from the sessions, coming as parents who were 'bringing' their child, focussed on their struggles as a parental couple. As I came to understand it, at least in part, their preoccupation with their son was both a defence against, and at times an expression of, the couple's core anxieties in their relationship. It was these anxieties that prevented them from coming together as a couple in order to support one another in being partners in parenting. Their initial position of psychic merger, and projective identification with their son, shifted as we were able to get hold of the unconscious phantasies around intimate relating and their anxieties about this started to be worked through.

More psychic separateness emerged as there was the beginning of a tolerance of greater intimacy within the couple, along with their developing a capacity to inhabit a 'third position' with one another, and with their son. It is this which, ultimately, unites the psychic worlds of parents and child, who are then held together in a 'triangular psychic space' in which there is room for both – establishing what Morgan (2005) has termed a 'creative couple relationship' which enables and supports creative and engaged parenting. The work I have described which focused on their anxieties about coupling was not 'instead of' addressing their parenting problems, but a necessary process of helping to establish a relationship in which the parents could function together as a creative parental couple.

I have sought to show how, whilst not focusing directly on strategies for improving parenting, couple therapy can help parents to establish a less defensive coupling, which at times excludes, and at others, includes, the children in a 'linked separateness' with them; the partners in the couple establishing a relationship with each other in which, in enabling intimacy between them, they can parent their children more freely. As a potential outgrowth of the therapeutic work, then, for couples with difficulties in this area of their psychic development, there may be a move towards a more mature experience of the Oedipus situation, whereby the parents establish a capacity for a 'third position', enabling their relationship to become a containing resource for them. This is of profound importance, not only for the stability and mental health of the adult couple, but for their children, and it is the significance of this for the psychic development of the child that DH Lawrence describes in this second quotation from his novel *The Rainbow* (cited by Clulow, 2019), where the emotional situation for the young girl, Anna, whom we met briefly earlier, has now changed as the parental couple relationship has developed:

> ***Anna's soul was at peace between them … .She was no longer called upon to uphold with her childish might the broken end of the arch. Her father and mother now met to the span the heavens, and she, the child, was free to play in the space beneath, between.***
> (The Rainbow (1915), p. 88)

This is a beautiful image of the child finding a place of freedom within the protective triangular space of the parental couple's relationship – so that she, the next generation, may grow emotionally and develop creative relationships of her own in times to come.

Disclosure statement

No potential conflict of interest was reported by the author(s).

References

Balfour, A. (2005). The couple, their marriage and oedipus. In F. Grier (Ed.), *Oedipus and the couple* (pp. 49-71). Karnac.

Balfour, A., Morgan, M., & Vincent, C. (Eds.). (2012). *How couple relationships shape our world. Clinical practice, research and policy perspectives*. Karnac.

Balfour, F., Clulow, C., & Dearnely, B. (1986). The outcome of maritally focussed psychotherapy as a possible model for marital psychotherapy outcome studies. *British Journal of Psychotherapy*, *3*(2), 133–143. https://doi.org/10.1111/j.1752-0118.1986.tb00964.x

Birkstead-Breen, D. (1996). Phallus, penis and mental space. *International Journal of Psychoanalysis*, *77*, 649–657.

Britton, R. (1989). The missing link: Parental sexuality in the Oedipus complex. In J. Steiner (Ed.), *The oedipus complex today: Clinical implications* (pp. 83-101). Karnac.

Clulow, C. (2019). Couples becoming parents. In A. Balfour, C. Clulow, and K. Thompson (Eds.), *Engaging couples: new directions in therapeutic work with families* (p. 41). Routledge.

Cowan, P., & Pape Cowan, C. (2009). Couple relationships: A missing link between adult attachment and children's outcomes. *Attachment & Human Development*, *11*(1), 1–4. https://doi.org/10.1080/14616730802500149

Glasser, M. (1979). Aggression and sadism in the perversions. In I. Rosen (Ed.), *Sexual deviation* (pp. 279-304). Oxford University Press.

Harold, G. T., & Leve, L. D. (2012). Parents as partners: How the parental relationship affects children's psychological development. In A. Balfour, M. Morgan, & C. Vincent (Eds.), *How couple relationships shape our world: Clinical practice, research and policy perspectives* (pp. 25-55). Routledge.

Harold, G. T., Pryor, J., & Reynolds, J. (2001). *Not in front of the children? How conflict between parents affects children*. One-Plus-One Marriage and Partnership Research.

Hewison, D., Casey, P., & Mwamba, N. (2016). The effectiveness of couple therapy: clinical outcomes in a naturalistic United Kingdom setting. *Psychotherapy*, *53*(4), 376. https://doi.org/10.1037/pst0000098

Klein, M. (1928). Early stages of the oedipus conflict. *International Journal of Psychoanalysis*, *9*, 167–180 (reprinted in *Love, Guilt and Reparation*. London: Hogarth Press, 1975).

Komaromi, T. (2019). *Childline annual review*. NSPCC. https://learning.nspcc.org.uk/media/1898/childline-annual-review-2018-19.pdf?_g...

Lawrence, D. H. (1915). *The rainbow*. Martin Secker, 1928.

Meier, R. (2018). *Addressing interparental conflict in child and adolescent mental health services*. Policy Briefing, Tavistock Relationships.

Morgan, M. (2001). First contacts: The therapist's 'couple state of mind' as a factor in containment of couples seen for consultations. In F. Grier (Ed.), *Brief encounters with couples: Some analytical perspectives* (pp. 17–32). Karnac.

Morgan, M. (2005). On being able to be a couple: The importance of a 'creative couple' in psychic life. In F. Grier (Ed.), *Oedipus and the couple* (pp. 9–30). Karnac.

Morgan, M. (2017). Unconscious beliefs about being a couple. In S. Nathans & M. Schaefer (Eds.), *Couples on the couch: Psychoanalytic couple psychotherapy and the Tavistock Model* (pp. 62–81). Routledge.

Rey, H. (1994). *Universals of psychoanalysis in the treatment of psychotic and borderline states*. Free Association Books.

Steiner, J. (1993). Problems of psychoanalytic technique: Patient-centred and analyst-centred interpretations. In *Psychic retreats: Pathological organisations in psychotic, neurotic and borderline patients* (pp. 131–146). Routledge.

Decolonising psychotherapy. Racism and the psychoanalytic profession

Helen Morgan

From time-to-time concern is expressed within the psychoanalytic community that so few individuals from the black and minority ethnic communities want to train with us and join our organisations. I have come to believe that these discussions many will be familiar with are not only futile but a part of the defensive structures that serve to act against the radical change that is needed. I know individuals change. However, apart from some tinkering, our institutions do not. This paper considers the defensive structures of disavowal within ourselves and our organisations as well as the features of psychoanalytic training that produce a disabling complacency. These work against the radical changes that are required if the profession is to become one to which people of colour can feel they belong and that reflects twenty first century multicultural Britain. I offer some suggestions for ways of working against the racist assumptions behind some of our theories and our structures. The underlying conviction of the presentation is that this is a white problem which white people need to address – not only for the benefit of black colleagues but because it also does us all harm.

Introduction

My first experience of a formal discussion about race and racism within the world of psychotherapy was in the 80's when, as a trainee, I attended a presentation by Lennox Thomas in my training organisation. Lennox was one of the first black people to train in psychoanalytic psychotherapy in Britain and became an important figure as a writer, teacher and activist.

The seminar I attended was around thirty-five years ago, but I still have memories of the evening. I came to London to train and was employed as a care worker in a Therapeutic Community for adults with mental health difficulties in North West London. There I met and worked with black colleagues and clients and was on a steep learning curve regarding racism – especially my own. Lennox's presentation, therefore, was very welcome. Throughout the talk

Lennox was controlled and gentle, taking care not to alienate his all white, mostly female audience. He drew comparisons with gender, speaking of his obligation as a man to be aware of, and think about, the female experience and to take responsibility for how his behaviour might impact on women. He was asking us, in turn, to take responsibility for our racism. Throughout the evening, he applied a solid understanding of psychoanalytic principles to make his case.

I was impressed and moved by the talk as he opened up connections between what I was learning in my training and my experiences at work and presented a whole new landscape I was keen to explore. Eagerly I waited for the discussion to see how others were affected and what my training organisation might consider doing in response. However, the conversation was deeply disappointing. No one directly challenged Lennox. No blatantly racist comment was made. Every speaker started with gratitude and an almost obsequious praise. Then each went on to make a comment that served to eradicate any possibility of potency from his talk. There was a series of personal statements from the audience, all of which asserted an exceptionalism that removed the speaker from the list of whites who might need to think about his words. Others asked why we were not discussing other injustices (class, gender, sexuality etc) managing to drown the matter of racism in a list of social wrongs. Further ‘questions’ were thinly disguised complaints that, really, it was all black people’s fault.

Over years of writing and speaking on the subject I have heard these ways we white people use to defend ourselves from thinking about our own racism many, many times. The list is depressingly limited, ubiquitous, and repetitive.

Since that evening I have tried to address the issue of racism from a number of positions within the profession. Starting as a young angry trainee, to writing and teaching as a more senior member of the profession, to becoming Chair of my own membership and training organisation, and then Chair of my regulatory body, the British Psychoanalytic Council. Working with colleagues we conducted research projects, set up working groups and conferences, raised matters at Council and called meetings of those responsible for training.

There has been some change. I used to experience outright hostility where students and course participants were openly angry that time had to be spent on this ‘irrelevant’ subject when they had so many other things to learn. People now are generally more open to the chance to focus on the problem and think about the implications for themselves and their work. I do know individuals change. However, apart from some tinkering, our institutions do not.

The experience of Black and Asian Minority Ethnic trainees

Black, Asian and Minority Ethnic people who have grown up in Britain, will have suffered from racism in some form or another; it will have been – and continues to be – a dimension of their personal and social life which needs acknowledgement and understanding. However, it is often reported by black psychotherapy students that their predominantly white analysts, supervisors and trainers mostly fail to recognise the reality of the problem. At best the consequence is that significant concerns and personal experiences are not thought about and understood within the ordinary analytic endeavour, or, at worst, previous trauma is repeated and reinforced.

In 2004, Margaret James-Franklin interviewed a number of black psychoanalytic psychotherapists who had trained in different psychotherapy organisations about their experiences for her MSc dissertation. Some years later a group of us in the (then) BAP carried out a survey across the organisation; the findings were written up by Karen Ciclitira and Nina Foster and published (Ciclitira & Foster, 2012). In 2013/2014 the Ethnicity, Culture and Racism Task Group of the British Psychoanalytic Council (BPC), chaired by Maxine Dennis, undertook a survey of registrants on attitudes to how ethnicity is addressed in their Member Institution. These findings were presented to an extended meeting of the senior leadership of the training organisations which are registered with the BPC.

What emerges from this research is how hard it is for the black individual to get through a training in psychoanalytic psychotherapy. The pressures are subtle but wearing. Some felt that their ethnicity attracted negative special attention during the interview process citing instances of being quizzed on matters not put to white applicants. Many spoke of raising questions and concerns in seminars about theoretical and clinical material from the point of view of diversity, racial difference, cultural variation, racism etc. which were ignored or dismissed by teachers and peers who were clearly uncomfortable in speaking freely about these issues. Many were told explicitly or implicitly that, because this was depth, analytic work, the difference in 'race' and colour was irrelevant. This leaves the black trainee in an invidious position. If they raise the issue they can be seen as being 'difficult' in bringing such uncomfortable matters into the room or failing to be sufficiently 'analytic' by focussing on so-called 'outer world' concerns. But if they don't speak then they collude with what amounts to a whitewash. Very few could recall times when the subject was raised by white seminar leaders, supervisors or colleagues.

Taken as a whole, the research reveals a climate of colour-blindness where trainers, supervisors and analysts take the position that differences in colour are not noticed and not relevant to in-depth, analytic work; we are assumed to all be the same. This denial of the reality of the impact of racism and power differentials means the black trainee is required to disregard important aspects of her or his experience and put aside their 'blackness' if they are to survive.

Frank Lowe (2006) writes:

> I haven't met a black therapist or trainee therapist who has been satisfied with their training organization's handling of race issues or feels confident that the profession is addressing the problem. I have explored how colour blindness or race avoidance can occur as a defence against fear and helplessness and I believe it also operates at

> an institutional level as a mechanism to maintain power, i.e. the status quo with its traditional power relations, authority and control. (p. 56)

He goes on to quote a number of black colleagues about their experience of training:

> 'Whenever I raise issues about race and culture, I am told this course is about the internal world not social issues' (Trainee child psychotherapist)
>
> 'During my interview I was asked about working with white patients but none of my fellow white trainees were asked about their ability to work with black patients.' (Adult psychotherapist)
>
> 'I feel isolated with my experience of the training and I do not feel confident that I will get support if I talk about my experience and views as a black person. I think it's probably best to just keep my head down and get through the training' (Trainee adult psychotherapist). (Lowe, 2006, p. 56-57)

Eugene Ellis is the founder and Director of the Black and Asian Therapy Network (BAATN). In an interview (Ellis, 2013) he points out:

> What tends to happen with Black trainees is that they enter into the spirit of enquiry that is encouraged on any counselling or psychotherapy training course, but when they do so in the area of their culture and their race, there is all this silence and it's like you've just opened a huge hole in the floor. Somehow it becomes your fault. You can then choose either to say nothing, because it's too painful, and focus on just getting your qualification, or you insist that your voice is heard, get labelled as the troublemaker, and risk not making it to the end because you're worn out by the fighting. It's so sad to see this happen and I have heard this from so many Black and Asian students. It all goes on under the surface. Just naming what's going on becomes almost impossible and everyone gets defensive and blaming. It's normally the student of colour who gets the rougher end of things because that's how oppression works. What then happens is that students have to go outside their training to get what they need to develop as therapists within the profession. (p. 16)

In a Working Note for a group interested in exploring matters of 'race' and equity in the profession, Andrew Cooper wrote the following:

> We think that for black and ethnic minority people the experience of racism tends to be pervasive in one form or another – but this does not mean that this is the whole of what their lives consist of! It is a dimension of personal and social experience. But a difficulty arises when they try to give voice to this aspect of their experience, because 'white' anglo-saxon people and institutions usually do not, or cannot, hear and simply take it seriously for what it is – one very important matter that needs understanding, recognition, and thought. We think the consequence of such a failure of response is predictable, and inevitable – a redoubled effort to make others 'take in' the seriousness of the issue, which can in turn lead to a more strenuous effort to renounce the (now even more) unpalatable communication. The stage is set for systematic misunderstanding and a culture of defensive 'race

> relations'- black people have a chip on their shoulder and white people are racist. (Internal BAP communication, July 2005)

A similar dynamic is described by Farhad Dalal (1998):

> What the marginalized groups are then forced to do, *as a strategic necessity*, is to ... assert an essentialism at the margins – the point about being at the margins is that the centre finds it hard to hear, partly because of psychological distance, and partly because what is being said is inconvenient. And so the marginalized are forced to shout until hoarse and can end up sounding shrill. (pp. 206–7, italics in original)

Disavowal of whiteness

Shannon Sullivan (2006) considers the trajectory of the great classical philosopher of race, W. E. B. Du Bois who began with:

> . . . .a "liberal" approach to the elimination of racism. Du Bois's liberalism naively posited human beings as always wishing to do good and as failing to do so only because they did not know what the good was . . . . Calling for white people to become more familiar with the lives and situations of black people, Du Bois put his faith in the basic goodness of white people. Their increased knowledge would reduce black people's (perceived) foreignness and eliminate the reason for white people's racist attitudes and behaviours towards them. (p. 20)

After World War I Du Bois went through a process of considerable disillusionment until he reached the position where he saw that:

> to understand the white ignorance of non-white people, one has to hear the active verb "to ignore" at the root of the noun. What had initially seemed to him like an innocent lack of knowledge on white people's part revealed itself to be a malicious production that masked the ugly Terrible of white exploitative ownership of non-white people and cultures. (Sullivan, 2006, p. 20)

In his autobiographical work, *Dusk of Dawn*, Du Bois (2007), writes:

> My own study of psychology under William James had pre-dated the Freudian era, but it had prepared me for it. I now began to realize that in the fight against race prejudice, we were not facing simply the rational, conscious determination of white folk to oppress us; we were facing age-long complexes sunk now largely to unconscious habit and irrational urge. (p. 148)

Psychoanalytic explanations of how racism operates tend to draw on the dynamics of projection, introjection and splitting. This helps to illuminate how the individual uses the system of racism that exists in society but it doesn't explain the system itself. Racism and the creation of the races is a social, political and economic phenomenon. It is a structure of power relations within which we live so the statement, 'I am not a racist,' is meaningless. Whilst it may be used by the individual psyche, that is not where the cause, nor the solution is located. A psychoanalytic approach can offer ways of thinking about how the system is maintained but we need to widen our thinking from the usual focus on the individual in isolation and see the connectivity between us. Farhad Dalal's concept of the social unconscious is helpful, as is that of the cultural complex and phantom narratives developed by the African American Jungian analyst, Sam Kimbles. The extension of the idea of the 'racial complex' has been taken up by Fanny Brewster in the US and Frank Lowe in the UK.

There is now plenty of research to show that children are aware of racism at a very early stage – as young as 3 or 4. It seems that the mechanism is a 'top-down' matter where, curious about the ways the world they have been born into is organised, they pick up the *fact* of power differentials and white privilege even if they don't yet understand the specific categories. The black child is likely to be surrounded by adults sufficiently resilient about discussing the concern to help them understand and manage what they are discovering about the world and their place in it.

However, white liberal parents are more likely to become embarrassed, hush the child, ignore or distract them or resort to the short-cut of colour blindness by insisting that everyone is the same and equal. Such an assertion is not only untrue and denies what the child has observed and experienced, by focusing on the universality of humans the message is conveyed that it is the *recognition* of difference that is the cause of racism rather than the fact that the child has been born into a social system that discriminates against certain groups which they need help to acknowledge, understand and begin to think through their responses.

Ryan Parker (2019) writes that, as a result:

> white children learn to disconnect – to stop thinking, to stop noticing, to stop linking reality and history, and to turn off their empathic curiosity and care. If allowed to develop this curiosity and care would cause problems for whiteness' power and the privileges it claims and protects, for it would result in recognition of reality, which eventually might lead to responsibility-taking and reparation . . . . (p. 8)

In most other aspects of her or his life, the child in a modern white liberal family can take their curiosity about the world to the significant adults in their life. For the majority of the time their experience will be of lively engagement, attention and interest. When they raise the matter of differences concerning race and ethnicity and they are responded to with the sterility of a blanket colour-blind position, the lively, engaged presence they had known previously disappears, and they are faced with a blankness, a shutting down and a silencing. There is a 'deadness' which relates to the subject and the child quickly learns that the topic is not welcome for discussion. Their curiosity and developing concern for others, their preoccupation with the troubled matter of social fairness is shut down and the vertical split of disavowal develops within the psyche.

In psychoanalytic theory, an internal conflict may lead to the creation of *horizontal* splits where aspects of the self are repressed, made unconscious and denied. Whilst also a defensive process, disavowal develops *within* the ego when it is faced with two conflicting realities causing a *vertical* split within the psyche. Unlike repression, the individual remains conscious of both sides of the split but will disavow either to meet internal desires and needs or minimise anxiety. Thus, I can know the reality of the consequences of my behaviour but will disregard that awareness in order to satisfy my desires, my omnipotence and my narcissistic sense of entitlement.

Disavowal for the white liberal splits the investment in white privilege together with its racist underpinning on one side and the need to maintain a sense of oneself as good on the other. Because of the numbing effect of colour-blindness, a void is created between the two, a silent gap, which lacks the capacity for mourning or symbolisation which Adrienne Harris (2012) – borrowing from Andre Green – calls a '*psychose blanche*'. Harris also takes Ruth Stein's concept of the *perverse pact* to suggest that such a contract operates unconsciously *between* white individuals and groups to ensure that white privilege is maintained whilst looking like work on change is taking place.

Racism and the profession

I had once assumed that the profession of psychoanalytic psychotherapy would be especially open to the challenge, as at our heart is a recognition and awareness of unconscious dynamics within the psyche that have a profound effect on our thoughts and action. I assumed we would be keen to understand our hidden racism and bring our analytic skills to the table in order to address the problem. I now believe that there are aspects of our thinking and our ways of training and structuring ourselves that contrive to ensure we convince ourselves that, really, there is no problem to address and that, if there is, then only some small adjustments are required. Thus we collude in what Bob Young (1994) describes as '*a loud silence*'.

Institutional racism

The Macpherson inquiry (1999) into the death of Stephen Lawrence defined institutional racism as:

> ... the collective failure of an organisation to provide an appropriate and professional service to people because of their colour, culture or ethnic origin. It can be seen or detected in processes, attitudes and behaviour which amount to discrimination through unwitting prejudice, ignorance, thoughtlessness and racist stereotyping which disadvantage minority ethnic people. (paragraph 6.34)

And: 'It is incumbent on every institution to examine their policies and the outcome of their policies and practices to guard against disadvantaging any section of our communities' (paragraph 46.27).

The psychoanalytic establishment is as susceptible to institutionalised racism as any other. However, the urgency and commitment that can be found in other professions such as social work, medicine, academia etc., is markedly lacking in that of ours. I don't think I have ever heard any blatantly racist statement made by a colleague – on the contrary, the language is usually of disapproval of racist dynamics within society. Most people I know are politically left of centre, many have worked in the public sector prior to training, and all express a concern for mental wellbeing throughout the population. And yet, as an institution there has been remarkably little real change.

Cooper (2018) writes:

> Institutional racism is both a manifestation of organizational resistance to change and a main source of that resistance. But tackling institutional racism is about the pursuit of ordinariness, about creating conditions wherein, at a minimum, organizations fully effect the ordinariness of a multi-ethnic society. ... within the multi-ethnic environments of today the fact that ... one can find organizational enclaves apparently almost untouched by these changes is surely evidence of something deeper and more troubling. Almost without exception, I suggest, the major institutions of psychoanalytic psychotherapy and psychotherapy training in this country are just such enclaves. (p. 101)

I mentioned above that there is a general silence in this profession regarding racism and a denial that we have a problem. This is not quite true as the matter *is* raised on an infrequent but regular basis. From time to time during gatherings of colleagues in committees, working groups, conferences etc., someone will point out the whiteness of most – if not all of the group. We all nod and agree the matter needs serious attention and there follows a discussion of what might be done. The conversation becomes increasingly desultory and fades away. Then the subject disappears from agendas altogether until, some months later, as if obeying an implicit rule, the subject will be raised again. We go round and round the same circle and effectively nothing changes. Ellis describes above the response should a black person persist beyond what seems to be the allotted time allowed for debate. If a white person does so, there is far less risk but there will be a general irritation and they are likely to be labelled – perhaps not as a troublemaker but as someone with a problem.

I cannot separate myself from this depressing procedure having played my part many times in these institutionalised practices, but I am coming to believe that these discussions are themselves part of a complicit, unconscious contract we are all engaged in to ensure against the radical change that is required. People feel caught in a Catch-22 of wanting to increase the diversity of the group, but the pool of available black colleagues is limited, and they can't be everywhere. Besides, there are worrying questions of tokenism, of looking to black people to save us whilst we assume a position of helplessness.

We have plenty of evidence open and available to us, both of the experience of black people in the profession and proposals for ways forward in the form of research reports, papers and articles. It seems we are unable to imagine questions we might ask ourselves, actions we might take, feelings we could explore and ways of doing so. Instead we are left in a state of apparent paralysis as if there is nothing to be done and, with apparent regret, (and a sigh of relief?) we move on

Robin DiAngelo (2018) notes that:

> To continue reproducing racial inequality, the system only needs white people to be really nice and carry on, smile at people of color, be friendly across race, and go to lunch together on occasions. I am not saying you shouldn't be nice. I suppose it's better than being mean. But niceness is not courageous. Niceness will not get racism on the table and will not keep it on the table when everyone wants it off. In fact, bringing racism to white people's attention is often seen as not nice, and being perceived as not nice triggers white fragility. (p. 153)

She suggests that

> Because White Fragility finds its support in and is a function of white privilege, fragility and privilege result in responses that function to restore equilibrium and return the resources "lost" via the challenge – resistance towards the trigger, shutting down and/or tuning out, indulgence in emotional incapacitation such as guilt or hurt feelings, exiting, or a combination of these responses. (p. 58)

White fragility is not weakness but a means of maintaining the privilege of whiteness. This fragility takes the form of colour-blindness that bypasses the realities of inequality and negates the need for engagement with the consequences of disparity and discrimination. This means we are unused to participating in ordinary conversations about the fact of that privilege and its implications. We have nothing like the resilience of black friends and colleagues with whom honest engagement becomes fraught with our anxiety, defensiveness and denial.

Discussions around racism in the profession often have a dead feel to them, as if we are going through the motions until, lacking libidinal investment, the conversation dribbles away and we can return to things as they were. I am coming to see such familiar discussions as a form of institutional ritual that acts to patch over the gap created by disavowal so that it is never properly faced and worked with. It serves the dual purpose of allowing us to feel we are doing something, that we are being nice, whilst actually ensuring that nothing really changes.

A problematic history

Both the theory and method of psychoanalysis and Jungian analysis contains an exasperating polarity that makes it both profoundly radical and also deeply conservative. As Stephen Frosh (2013) puts it: 'This ambiguity inherent in psychoanalysis infects everything it comes into contact with. Both conformist and revolutionary, both racist and emancipatory, it shows how we are continuously infiltrated by things we know little about, or that we thought we had escaped' (p. 9).

Gilman (1993) points out that, at the time when Freud and his followers were working on this new theory in Vienna, Jews were thought of as 'blacks' and, therefore, psychoanalysis, as a 'black thing' (pp. 121–122). At the start, the project developed at the margins of society and spoke its radical message from this position. As Freud and his followers left Germany and Austria and moved elsewhere, they needed to fit in, find acceptance and establish a place within the privileged world of the white middle classes of the UK and the Americas. The price of this contract was the omission of race and social class from its discourse and consequently the increased homogeneity of its members such that today, looking around most gatherings of psychoanalytic psychotherapists, one could be forgiven for thinking that psychoanalysis has now become a 'white thing': 'When a black thing turns into a white thing, we might well wonder what processes of disavowal and repression are at work' (Gilman, 1993, p. 122).

Neil Altman states:

> As a black thing in a white society, psychoanalysis attained the power of the outsider to gain perspective to critique, to see in the dark. A large share of the value of psychoanalysis derives from the ability of Freud and his followers to bring to light that which was disavowed and repressed. In becoming white in America, psychoanalysts forfeited some of that night vision, most particularly with respect to our own social (meaning racial and class) position and the ways this process might be reflected in clinical work. The position we have on the polarity is reversed, but the polarity remains. And so we find ourselves needing and resisting the critique, the psychoanalytic intervention, of those we have left out. (Altman, 2010, p. 123)

Altman's (2010) book is called *The Analyst in the Inner City*. He points out that 'Historically, psychoanalysis has largely eschewed concern with inner-city public clinic work .... Psychoanalysts concentrated on private practice, where conditions more neatly fitted the classical ideal and where, not incidentally, there was more money to be made.' (p. xv). The British psychoanalyst Harvey Taylor (2013) in his discussion paper notes that:

> ... at the 1918 Budapest international conference Freud and the early pioneers agreed that psychoanalysis would develop along three fronts: research, training and subsidised clinics. Owing to inflation and political developments in Eastern Europe only the training option was developed, supported by a limited research effort based on the case history. (p. 2–3)

The abandonment of the subsidised clinic and of the discourse around race and class has deprived the discipline of a width of human experience and narrowed the field of knowledge. There are those in the psychoanalytic community who, like Altman, work in public health settings, in prisons, working-class community projects, with the homeless and the poor, and have first-hand experience of the impact of social injustice and oppression on the individual and the family. Yet they have little say in the formulation of our clinical theory. We rarely hear case presentations involving shop assistants, migrant workers, lorry drivers, or care workers. Jennifer Tolleson (2009), in her ironically titled paper 'Saving the World One Patient at a Time' notes that 'Working from the margins, these clinicians have contact with our culture's hidden subjectivities ... (which) ... comprise hidden – subjugated – knowledges that remain, sadly, outside our formidable intelligence as a profession (pp. 201–202).

The radical potential of psychoanalysis is expressed by Harris (2012) who asserts that:

> … .the method of psychoanalysis … . is a commitment to looking at both what is hidden in silence and in plain sight. Psychoanalysis, at its most unflinching and courageous, allows us to maintain curiosity at the strange, fuzzy, unreasoning moments in the psyche and in the culture. In this way, psychoanalysis has the potential to be, in part, a revolutionary practice. Or to put it more modestly, psychoanalysis can be part of a radical practice of social resistance. (p. 198)

However, the conservative pull resists taking on the revolutionary implications of our understanding when it comes to developing and supporting a radical practice in relation to race. Melanie Suchet (2007) writes:

> … within psychoanalysis the place of race in the construction of subjectivity has always been minimized. A curious omission given that formation of the subject is our field of study. Discussions of race today remain largely limited to an investigation of otherness when someone of a different color enters the consulting room. Further, the burden of writing about race has until very recently fallen on those with darker skins who have been trying to tell us for decades that a racialized subjectivity is crucial. (p. 868)

'Inner' and 'outer'

Our theories presume and perpetuate a division between 'inner' and 'outer', between the 'psyche' and the 'social' where the former is considered the proper subject for psychoanalysis. This can lead to an assumption, not always explicit, that injustices such as racism are 'outer', social world phenomena therefore, of little or no relevance to analytic enquiry. Traditionally our theories isolate the individual from their social world, and we prioritise the personal over the political although recent developments such as relational psychoanalysis seek to re-instate the link. Dalal (2002) challenges the assumptions behind the usual psychoanalytic perspectives which he sees as locating the *cause* of racism as an internal world dynamic rather than in the social world. He says: 'In my opinion, the problems thrown up in this territory shed light on a more general difficulty in psychoanalytic theories; a difficulty born of a false distinction between the *developmental* and *socialization* processes' (p. 80; italics in the original).

In academia there is a debate about the validity of any division between the internal and the external and the implications of isolating one from the other. Stephen Frosh and Baraitser (2008) for example, argue that:

> The division is . . . a way of doing politics, and the psycho-social becomes a contrary way of doing politics, a rebellion that asserts that you cannot have one without the other, that they are warp and weft and signifier and signified, and so on through the different ways of saying that they are two sides of the same thing. (p. 349)

In his response to this paper, Paul Hogget (2008) takes issue with the idea that the distinction should be dissolved entirely asserting a *belief* 'that the internal and external worlds, while overlapping and mutually constituting, are also irreducible to one another. Each is governed by its own rules of structure formation. (p. 383).

I came across this intriguing and thought-provoking debate within psycho-social studies in my research for the book. It struck me that our profession ought to be more actively involved in the conversation both because of what we might contribute and what we could learn. It was not the first time I stumbled on a perspective from outside of the world of clinicians that challenged a set of age-old assumptions and woke up my thinking. It underlined how insulated we are from other disciplines. In our conferences, seminars and journals we tend to talk mostly to ourselves generally confirming or expanding slightly what we already know. It seems we are missing out on a world of thinking and debate which we might find stimulating, original and helpful for we could do with collapsing a little the old categories of the individual and the social, the internal and the external and find better ways of theorising how human suffering can be both personal *and* collective.

Complacency

To turn to the libraries of other specialties – even those who are our friends – requires a certain humility which I fear can be lacking in our world. Doubtless all disciplines have their certainties but ours seems particularly prone to complacency. There is a tendency – possibly exacerbated by external attack – towards a position of arrogance where our theories are spoken as if they were 'the truth'. Sometimes when we take psychoanalytic thinking out into society, we do so as if we bring a golden thing for which the world should be grateful. A humility is required of us, one that recognises we too have much to learn. To borrow from Bion: 'Psychoanalysis is just one stripe on the coat of the tiger' (Bion, 1991).

Frosh and Baraitser (2008) again:

> . . . many psychosocial researchers share the traditional sociological suspicion of psychoanalysis because of its strong individualizing tendencies, while those who have been most influenced by poststructuralist and/or discursive perspectives resist

> the 'top-down' expert-knowledge epistemological strategies of psychoanalysis with their apparent certainties about the 'true' nature of human subjectivity, accompanied by an interpretive practice that always seems to know best, or at least to know subjects better than they know themselves. (p.347)

The myth of 'the complete analysis'

I wonder if one of the strengths of our craft – the fact that all psychoanalytic psychotherapists are required to be in analysis throughout our trainings – might also be a weakness. Perhaps there is a tendency to an unconscious – even conscious – belief in what I have come to think of as the myth of the complete analysis which leads to complacency as if we somehow have things more or less sorted. This is particularly dangerous when talking about race. Given most white members have had analysis with a white analyst I suspect the analysand will not have spent many sessions exploring their racism. Certainly, I don't recall the subject ever coming up in mine. Yet I am often surprised by the certainty I meet in individuals as if there really is nothing further that needs consideration or thought about oneself.

Ways forward

There are many thoughtful, socially concerned and politically aware people within the profession who are troubled by injustice and discriminatory practices and are genuine in their wish to make a difference. But we work against deep conscious and unconscious dynamics that operate in ourselves as individuals and in our institutions and we need to recognise and be careful of these undercurrents and their effects if we are to take on the hard work that is needed if real change is to come about. I suggest the usual discussions that many will be familiar with are not only futile but are a part of the defensive structures that serve to act against the radical change that is needed. If such structures are there to defend our white privilege, then radical change will require acknowledgement of that privilege and letting it go. There will be loss and discomfort, but I argue that our liberal, justice and knowledge seeking concerned selves will gain immeasurably.

The following are just some ideas of how we might take this work forward.

Action

(1) A radical review of the theories we use through a series of reading groups and group discussions. There is a paucity of material within the analytic texts that offers a thorough critique of the colonial roots of some of the terms we use and we will need to borrow heavily from those in academia such as psycho-social studies, philosophy and social work. There are colleagues in these departments who understand and are sympathetic to psychoanalytic theory but have also researched and written about the more questionable history and modern-day implications. Recently in my own organisation, the British Jungian Analytic

Association (BJAA) within the BPF, groups of us have met to explore potentially troubling concepts such as the 'primitive', 'inner and outer' and the more Jungian concepts of 'animus/anima' and '*participation mystique*'. For each meeting we read two papers on the topic – usually from contrasting perspectives – and then met to discuss. According to the responses from those involved, this has led to an organic re-vision of these concepts and a re-think of the way we work and teach. Certainly, the energy generated has been in considerable contrast with the flat, deadly discussions we usually have about racism, gender and sexuality. I gather that the words 'critique' and 'crisis' have a common etymological origin. Certainly members of the group reported a sense a crisis of thought in this process of critiquing long accepted, previously unquestioned theories, but most seemed to feel it was a crisis worth weathering.

(2) A greater vigilance regarding language and text is required. The writings of our analytic forbears, sadly especially Jung, is peppered with assumptions, pronouncements and language which is ugly and abusive .... As a white analyst, teacher and supervisor, it is *my* responsibility to see and to question and be disturbed by the disturbing and questionable material. I need to imagine what it might feel like to have one's ancestors referred to as 'savage' or primitive' .... Either I must leave such texts off the reading list or I must introduce them in a manner that acknowledges the hurt they may cause and open up and facilitate a conversation about the implications. This must be done whether there is a black person present or not. For if we train white analysts to believe there is nothing to notice, nothing to be concerned about, then the abuse continues, and we cripple the future growth of therapists.

(3) From an organisational perspective, a thorough evaluation of all aspects of its life from monitoring systems, policies, structures etc needs to be undertaken by each training and/or membership or regulatory body. Frank Lowe (2006) writes:

> There must be a systematic review of analytic organizations' ways of functioning, in terms of whether and how they disadvantage black and minority communities. This would include the selection of psychotherapists for training, content of training programmes and supervision arrangements. Overall, this is about changing organizational culture and developing a non-defensive but non-persecutory approach to exploring racism rather than avoidance, denial and splitting it off from awareness at the intra-psychic, interpersonal, group and organizational levels. (p. 49-50)

(4) This requirement on organisations must include our regulatory bodies such as the BPC, the UKCP and the BACP. Accurate and thoughtful monitoring of the make-up of the profession needs to be undertaken to give a clear and up to date picture of the demography of the profession. Questions of how each organisation and each member is actively addressing development towards tackling racism needs to be a key aspect of all

elements of the regulatory process including ethics, CPD requirements and registration of member institutions.

(5) We can utilise ways familiar to us such as seminars, scientific meetings and conferences for deepening our understanding of how racism operates. I suggest we also need to explore the live intra- and inter-psychic emotional processes of racism. White privilege is deep-rooted and not always visible to white people or accessible to a psychoanalytic approach. An understanding of how it works, how it might be given up and the subsequent costs (and benefits) for those identified as white requires creative approaches which can reach beyond the intellect is essential if there are to be genuine and effective changes. Experiential groups, affinity groups, social dreaming, group analytic events are the sort of methods which may be helpful as ways to bypass the intellectualising defenses. Such endeavours need support from organisations and the experiences written up and shared through publication in newsletters, journals etc. It is important to hold in mind that the radical/conservative binary that runs as a thread through our theory and practice also runs through us as organisations, groups and individuals. We need to stay alert to the splitting of the binary, where we each take up one of the polarised positions and deny and disown the opposite. This will lead again to organisational stuckness. We might need external support and consultancy to help us with this.

Endnote

Joel Kovel (1988) uses the term 'saturate' to describe the way in which racism has penetrated every corner of the society into which we are all born. There is no position one can take which is outside it. If we acknowledge the racist backdrop to our world then we also have to recognise the particular prejudicial veil which is the inheritance of all white members of this society. The veil may well be one of cordiality, but it has guilt, shame and envy woven into it which freezes our curiosity about each other and prevents us from having ordinary conversations about the realities of the impact of racism.

In his book *Partisans in an Uncertain World*, Paul Hoggett says:

> .... *uncritical thought will not simply be passive but will actively cling to a belief in the appearance of certain things. It actively refuses, rejects as perverse or crazy, any view that may contradict it. To think critically one must therefore be able to use aggression to break through the limitations of one's own assumptions or to challenge the "squatting rights" of the colonizer within one's own internal world.* (Hoggett, 1992, p. 29)

Given the fact of global colonisation by white western culture, for us who are defined as belonging to such a culture, we can, if we choose, avoid external pressure to make that act of aggression that challenges the 'squatting rights' of the internal coloniser. But not noticing this figure who inhabits at least a corner of our minds demanding compliance does not mean he does not exist. I suggest that we are the poorer if we do not attempt the act of aggression to break through our assumptions for they then remain an area of psychic life that is unexamined. The stubbornness of the uncritical thought that actively clings to a belief in the appearance of certain things in Hoggett's quote may give us a clue to the tenacity of the fact of racism despite our wish that it were not so. For me to think differently about my place in the world and the privileges it has brought me requires an undoing of a well-laid system of assumptions about myself. The fact that those assumptions existed and continue to exist does not make me an inherently bad person, but to break through their limitations is hard work. This is not an easy subject to 'play' with. It raises feelings of guilt, shame, envy, denial and defiance, all of which are hard enough to face in the privacy of one's own life. To explore it publicly can bring up a fear of getting it wrong, of saying the unforgivable and of exposing an internal badness.

When white people choose to stay blind, deaf and silent concerning our own privilege and its impact on the black 'Other', we are opting to remain unconscious of a crucial aspect of our lives and of ourselves. This part of our shadow has been whitewashed out of view, but then what colours, what potential, what depth might we be missing?

I recall seeing a poster once, many years ago. A white man was being carried on a black man's back who was weighed down with his burden. The text gave the white man's words which went something like: '*I will care for you, empathise with you, weep for you for the load you have to carry. One thing I won't do is get off your back.*' There is no doubt that the greater suffering is shouldered by the black man, but the picture is not a healthy one for either. We white people need to climb down, stand on our own two feet and walk – for the sake of justice, but also for our own health, our own individuation, our own peace of mind.

Disclosure statement

No potential conflict of interest was reported by the author(s).

References

Altman, N. (2010). *The analyst in the inner city. Race, class and culture through a psychoanalytic lens*. Routledge.

Bion, W. R. (1991). *A memoir of the future*. Karnac.

Ciclitira, K., & Foster, N. (2012). Attention to culture and diversity in psychoanalytic trainings. *British Journal of Psychotherapy*, *28*(3), 353–373. https://doi.org/10.1111/j.1752-0118.2012.01298.x

Cooper, A. (2018). Institutional racism: Can our organizations change? In *Conjunctions. Social work, psychoanalysis and society* (pp. 99–116). Routledge .

Dalal, F. (1998). *Taking the group seriously: Towards a post-foulkesian group analytic theory*. Jessica Kingsley Publishers.

Dalal, F. (2002). *Race, colour and the process of racialization: New perspectives from group analysis, psychoanalysis and sociology*. Brunner Routledge.

DiAngelo, R. (2018). *White fragility. Why it's so hard for white people to talk about racism*. Penguin Random House.
Du Bois, W. E. B. (2007). *Dusk of dawn*. Oxford University Press. (First published by Harcourt, Brace and World Inc., 1940).
Ellis, E. (2013). *Silenced: The black student experience*. www.therapytoday.netTherapyTodayDecember
Frosh, S., & Baraitser, L. (2008). Psychoanalysis and psychosocial studies. *Psychpoanalysis, Culture & Society*, *13*(4), (346–365. https://doi.org/10.1057/pcs.2008.8
Frosh, S. (2013). *Hauntings: Psychoanalysis and ghostly transmissions*. Palgrave Macmillan.
Gilman, S. (1993). *Freud, race and gender*. Princeton University Press.
Harris, A. (2012). The house of difference, or white silence. *Studies in Gender and Sexuality*, *13*(3), 197–216. https://doi.org/10.1080/15240657.2012.707575
Hogget, P. (2008). What's in a hyphen? Reconstructing psychosocial studies. *Psychoanalysis, Culture & Society*, *13*(4), 379–384. https://doi.org/10.1057/pcs.2008.26
Hoggett, P. (1992). The art of the possible. In *Partisans in an uncertain world: The psychoanalysis of engagement* (pp. 10–39). Free Association Books.
Kovel, J. (1988). *White racism. A psychohistory*. Free Association Books.
Lowe, F. (2006). Racism as a borderline issue: The avoidance and marginalization of race in psychotherapy. In A. Foster, A. Dickenson, B. Bishop, & J. Kleine (Eds.), *Difference: An avoided topic in practice* (pp. 43–60). Karnac.
Macpherson, W. (1999). *The Stephen Lawrence Inquiry*. https://assets.publishing.service.gov.uk/government/uploads/system/uploads/attachment_data/file/277111/4262.pdf
Parker, R. N. (2019). Slavery in the white psyche. *Psychoanalytic Social Work*, *26*(1), 84–103. https://doi.org/10.1080/15228878.2019.1604240
Suchet, M. (2007). Unravelling whiteness. *Psychoanalytic Dialogues*, *17*(6), 867–886. https://doi.org/10.1080/10481880701703730
Sullivan, S. (2006). *Revealing whiteness. The unconscious habits of racial privilege*. Indiana University Press.
Taylor, H. 2013. *UK psychoanalysis: Mistaking the part for the whole*. British Psychoanalytic Council Discussion Paper.
Tolleson, J. (2009). Saving the world one patient at a time: Psychoanalysis and social critique. *Psychotherapy and Politics International*, *7*(3), 190–205. https://doi.org/10.1002/ppi.200
Young, R. (1994). Projective space: The racial other. In *Mental space* (pp. 93–119). Process Press.

Pandemic: challenges in care and recovery

Dinesh Sinha

Our experiences through the pandemic have to be viewed by reflecting on the year and a half that has been, but also what we have learnt through this experience, with a view to taking forward. The article intends to approach this topic, from a health and social care perspective coming from the author working in The Tavistock and Portman NHS Foundation Trust, a healthcare organisation, but also importantly, from a relational perspective in how we interact organisationally, as a health & social care system that is part of a wider society in this city, across the UK and the wider world.

The article not only comments on systemic inequalities that have become stark in the pandemic, but also identifies corrosive and deliberate counter narratives to the themes of care and courage in this period. It concludes that the pre-existing silos of separation between the privileged and dispossessed have prevented survival and wellbeing in the wider society.

The process of recovering from the pandemic is not just about the restoration of physical wellbeing but also the creation of healthier conditions in society that actively vitiate against the scourge of everyday sadism.

This has clearly been a time of extreme challenge, in particular (when I think back to March 2020) due to the unanticipated and frightening nature of the Covid 19 pandemic, as it unfolded with all its impact. Most of us will know someone who has been affected by the destruction and death from this terrible illness. We learnt the costly impact of ignoring the terrible infection that was sweeping nation after nation and of the families, who died looking after each other, successively catching a little understood contagion, as it wreaked havoc and caused repeated cycles of death. I remember in those first few months, when we struggled to understand the nature of the virus and how it affected attempts to live a normal day-to-day existence, while seeking to manage the impact at social and community levels of not being able to come together. The need for physical distancing felt really as if we were being asked to break up our cultural and social groups, both in our personal lives and at work.

The successive waves since the start last year have given more experience and opportunity to respond proactively, though there continue to be repeated instances of shock, trauma and exhaustion, due to the continuing litany of losses starting with things that we could no longer do in life, growing to the burdens of enforced distancing and finally the impact of illness and death, as it mounted over the past year and a half. What became clear is that the usual pigeon holes between the personal and professional, health systems and their social contexts, prevention and ill health to name a few, have become unhelpful and not aided the promotion of population health.

Society and its leadership's impact on healthcare in society

Over this period, generations have been left marked by the vagaries of the pandemic; which has continued in various parts of the world. The impact includes every age group, including people with more experience of life who have been left unsure and vulnerable, unable to seek the usual supports that keep them going, working adults who were left bereft of economic opportunities necessary to make something of their lives, and increasingly children and young people who have been unable to keep up with their education or have the normal range of development and stimulation, which is so crucial at these stages of life. Even with the knowledge that we were getting from other countries, there remain questions about how exactly the virus originated, where did it come from, how it become so pathogenic, all linked around wanting to understand with some transparency the causation of illness, which could lead to a range of treatment measures or even a cure.

This unknown virus and its consequent pandemic has followed the pattern of a highly infectious disease and in doing so, connected with what we know from the past, such as the well-recognised story of cholera spreading from a well in London.

'In the Victorian period the "miasmatic" theory of disease causation' was largely supported in preference of other modes of causation of illness, such as that proposed by John Snow. Dr Snow's 'hypothesis of polluted water being a cause of cholera was not accepted' . . . though he did eventually persuade the local parish to remove a water pump handle after noting 'the high incidence of mortality' (Halliday, 2001).

Unfortunately, our social responses have also often been fuelled by a similar deficit in knowledge and driven by fear and modern superstition.

Systems that were meant to be prepared

Certainly in the time since the first wave, there has been genuine perplexity and consternation here in the UK, across Europe and the rest of the world about systems that were meant to be prepared for just such an eventuality, for example EPRR (emergency preparedness resilience and response) in the NHS, PHE (Public Health England) and local authorities. Sadly, 'readiness' does not seem to have been borne out in the statistics of gross morbidity and mortality.

Freiden (2021) reported that Taiwan was the first nation to implement proactive measures against the novel Coronavirus. On 31 December 2019, Taiwan was the first nation to inform the World Health Organization of the potential for human-to-human transmission. Wuhan, China, started on-board health inspection of flight passengers from Wuhan to Taiwan. The use of innovative information technology, as critical steps in controlling the spread of Covid-19: contact-tracing, testing and quarantine or isolation-treatment. Common factors for success in such countries were openness to clinical/ scientific expertise by leadership, early shutdown, aggressive monitoring and a disciplined population.

In the UK, over the period of the pandemic, the Government has reported over 10 million cases and over 170,000 deaths that are recognised with Covid 19 on death certificates (253.4/100,000 population) (Gov.uk, 2021) though there is an ongoing debate regarding the accuracy of figures (Dyer, 2021). Perhaps then unsurprisingly, for patients and staff in healthcare, the impact of the pandemic has been enormous and in many instances catastrophic. A systematic review done after the peak of the first wave determined that a total of 152,888 infections and 1413 deaths were reported with more deaths in men and doctors (Bandyopadhyay et al., 2020). There have been numerous instances of trauma to entire familial generations. Meanwhile, deaths that till very recently were in thousands in this country on a weekly basis and continue in other parts of the world.

The calls for a public enquiry in England have finally been conceded, as examples have become far more visible of societies and countries that have done better, with similar challenges through the pandemic. The challenge for the upcoming enquiry is to respond to the questions of known and unknown gaps; who did what and when that may help clear our collective confusion of what part of this pandemic and its consequences were avoidable.

Care and commitment

The stories of commitment and courage, such as in health services, have been repeated through this period. There was and remains something very pure, unadulterated and inspiring in the individual and collective examples of this clarity of purpose towards the preservation of life, which gathered pace in the weeks after the first wave commenced and have continued ever since.

After the first few weeks of perplexity, there was the full embrace in the UK of innovation, collaboration and courage across health and social care settings, accompanied by numerous examples of staff and organisations working across boundaries to keep the system open and allow patients access to the care they needed.

Like other healthcare organisations, the Tavistock and Portman NHS Foundation Trust also embraced innovation and became a model of cross system working, in ways that we would never have even contemplated a year ago; for example, in delivering a significant proportion of our services through hybrid methods, ensuring the quality of care and continuing our role in promoting wellbeing and debate, such as through centenary events that attracted more than 7,000 staff, students, service users and the general public.

A corrosive counter narrative

However, when we look back it would be remiss to not also reflect on an equal and opposite reaction to the pandemic, in various forms that has continued through this period as a counter narrative to the theme of visible care and courage, such as in healthcare settings. There has been a corrosive counter narrative in almost every society, presenting in various guises. Arguments of economic growth versus population wellbeing being the basis for not implementing safety measures such as lockdowns or personal freedom of choice as a reason to not wear masks; progressing to outright lies, fake news culminating in exhortations challenging fact and science, often by population influencers, leaders and individuals. Themes have included questions about the existence of Covid 19, the use and benefits of masks, lockdowns, so called dangers of vaccines and beyond that baiting and gas lighting of populations on race and gender.

Some time ago, I spoke at an event on the quality of generosity and care for others being based in the capacity for gratitude; essentially that giving comes from being thankful from having received care. In contrast, what has been particularly concerning through the pandemic has been the rise of a number of instances that are not about offering care, but the very opposite and far, far beyond micro-aggressions. These splits could be understood as close to a societal manifestation of the paranoid-schizoid position described by Klein (1946). She progressed greatly an understanding of the early management of anxiety by the splitting of both self and object into good and bad. 'As a result, the breast, in as much as it is gratifying, is loved and felt to be "good"; in so far as it is a source of frustration, it is hated and felt to be "bad".' (Klein, 1997, p. 62). This early stage is universally developmental and is characterised by the use of splitting to manage contradictory feelings towards the same object, but can persist into more pathological states characterised by a lack of capacity for holding of ambivalence between persecution and idealisation even in adults.

This polarity and inflexible separateness lends itself to the patterns of significant splits in societal responses to the pandemic and primitive efforts to deal with *life threatening* persecutory anxieties. These are concretely evident in the lies in fake news, the challenging of fact and science, whether on social media, sensationalist news headlines or from thought leaders and influences. These have been disparate but related actions, that seem to have several common goals, including to confuse the reader, misinform, mislead and finally go in the opposite of the direction of care and preservation of life. What we see instead in the pandemic counter narrative is a pleasure in cruelty and a wish to profit from others misery.

In broader psychiatric thinking, such as embodied in the ICD 11 (international classification of diseases), the current diagnosis for sadism is limited to Coercive Sexual Sadism Disorder, which is defined as 'characterised by a sustained, focused and intense pattern of sexual arousal – as manifested by persistent sexual thoughts, fantasies, urges or behaviours – that involves the infliction of physical or psychological suffering on a non-consenting person. In addition, in order for Coercive Sexual Sadism Disorder to be diagnosed, the individual must have acted on these thoughts, fantasies or urges or be markedly distressed by them. Coercive Sexual Sadism Disorder specifically excludes consensual sexual sadism and masochism' (WHO, 2019).

However, there has been significant exploration of sadism in psychoanalytical thinking, starting with a theory of sadism and masochism, as innate drives by Freud and linked with his eventual exploration of the life and death drive. Ellis (1898–1928/1936) differed in that for him sadism and masochism were related and complementary forms of behaviour. Later, the core complex by Glasser mapped out the impact of missteps in ordinary development, if the anxieties of engulfment and separation become unmanageable. According to Glasser (1988), the core complex underpins paedophilia and all other perversions, which are driven by the urge to hurt the object. The core complex identified the use of sexualised aggression in managing primitive anxieties, such as of being engulfed by the object on one hand, while on the other the catastrophe of abandonment. In this way, he described the role of eroticisation in being employed to manage hate and the primitive need to destroy the object, which was then manifested in sadistic and masochistic behaviours. It is likely that a predisposition in sub sections of populations to the use of primitive defences, especially when faced with unmanageable anxiety, is linked to expressions of sadism and cruelty in societal forums.

Further insights come from the psychoanalytically based work on attachment and the development of personality. Meloy and Gacono (1998) described pathologies of attachment including fearful, preoccupied, disorganized and dismissive attachments. Dismissive attachment patterns have been linked with risk of violent offending (Fonagy, 1999) while 'chronic emotional detachment, cortical under arousal and minimal anxiety biologically anchor the foundation of the house of psychopath' as described by Meloy & Sheva (2007). There has been further work on the relationship between sadism and perversion in the work of various others including Benvenuto (2016), who linked sadism with resentment at its core. In his view, the perverse individual has the need to violate innocence by choosing to subject the other to humiliation, pain, disgust, and suffering. In this way, enjoyment of the suffering of the other forms a key part of sadism.

A few years ago, the concept of everyday sadism emerged, which seems an extension of earlier psychoanalytical and psychological models of sadism. There were links demonstrated by O'Meara and Hammond (2016) between the presence of psychopathic traits, social adaptation, such as being able to influence others and success in exploitation of others. This work resulted in the definitions of sadism being extended as a broader range of issues, as part of the dark tetrad of personality difficulties, to essentially indicate 'a preference for causing pain, humiliation and discomfort to others for pleasure, which is not necessarily sexual'. Indeed, the manifestation of sadism is in interpersonal spaces where the suffering may be physical, psychological or emotional, and so beyond only sexual expressions of sadism. Meere and Egan (2017) wrote that research on socially aversive personalities showing sadists willing to work for the opportunity to hurt an innocent person. In their work, sadism emerged as an independent predictor of behaviour reflecting an appetite for cruelty. Hence, it is possible to draw relationships between patterns of particular relational pathologies and the narrative of cruelty observed in this pandemic. In such a social and political context, there is an automatic negation of the need for care, such as what happened to the doctor who died raising the fact about the virus.

His words in a final interview were powerful 'The police believed this virus was not confirmed to be SARS. They believed I was spreading rumours. They asked me to acknowledge that I was at fault. I felt I was being wronged, but I had to accept it. Obviously I had been acting out of *good* will. I felt very sad seeing so many people losing their loved ones' (Hegarty, 2020). Examples have included a president who told his people they need 'to stop whining' after over a quarter of a million deaths in that country! A mayor from the same geography asked people to sacrifice themselves for the economy by going out to work without masks; another president who told others to inhale herb infused smoke and not do lockdowns; all active exhortations to disregard knowledge and spread rumours and hatred.

What does the wealth of society do for its people? The questions that do arise from such examples suggest a relationship between a certain kind of societal contract and its reflected leadership, which go to the core of a collective understanding (or its lack of) between wellbeing and ill health, regardless of the leaning of the government. In this fervid context, there has been a potent and dangerous mix of health, business and politics prioritising arguments of economic growth versus population health. It is perhaps no surprise that the people, who are particularly opposed to the facts of the infection and need for protection/vaccination, are also particularly bellicose about the need for economic activity. Unsurprisingly, they are often also the wealthiest, who are able to protect themselves from exposure to the virus and have access to the best medical care, if unwell.

Further inequalities

Oxygen and its deprivation is a frequent theme in this pandemic, such as when Covid-19 stops it from being absorbed by the lungs or its lack as a treatment in short supply kills from asphyxiation. It features also in the counter narrative, when it is deliberately withheld, such as from a knee on the windpipe and in this brutal act exposes long known multiple generational and systemic inequalities.

Hutchinson (2020) reported that a doctor died in the US 'described how her pain had been downplayed by the doctor, whom she said was white, though she had been crying and having difficulty breathing'. 'He did not even listen to my lungs; he didn't touch me in any way. He performed no physical exam. I told him you cannot tell me how I feel'. This experience was in the context of well-known concerns in that country on the racial/ethnic bias among Health Care Professionals and its influence on health care outcomes (Hutchinson, 2020). There is further data from the US suggesting that ethnically diverse people living in more densely populated areas, having to use public transport and working in low paid service jobs, such as without sick pay meant that people from these populations are more likely to end up with increase in the risk of exposure to the virus. These populations have been known to have a higher rate of cardiac disease, diabetes and hypertension, which all are also known to be linked with social inequalities (Kirby, 2020). Nearer home, an IFS (Institute of Fiscal Studies) review by Platt and Warwick (2020) found a much higher rate of death, particularly black African populations within the ethnically diverse group, after removing impact of role and geography, as having something like a 3.7 times more likelihood to die than white British population.

All this suggests that those amongst us who have been the most vulnerable pre pandemic have been the worst affected. It would not be too great an extrapolation to hold concern about their ability to recover even to their pre pandemic states in the coming period.

The future and what it means for us

'You never make change by fighting the existing reality. To change something, build a new model that makes the existing model obsolete' (R. Buckminster Fuller)

The pandemic has not ended and on an individual level for healthcare staff, the year and a half mark will be a harsh milestone, but also one that offers salutary lessons. It has made more evident our innate capacity for resilience and courage that we may have previously been unaware of to such a degree. However, there are aspects of what we are left with that remain concerning, such as feeling traumatised, exhausted and angry, even as we face the prospect of another harsh winter.

How do we care for our needs in order to retain our capacity to care for others? There remain tensions in properly attending to work versus just being present. This while also dealing with exhaustion and guilt of having survived when thousands of our colleagues in the frontlines have not. It makes it an even greater need to not forget those who have lost their lives while at work in health, so we don't lapse into masochism and bravery, which would lead to the fraying of our professional stance and the work of recovery that confronts us all. We must be aware of and seek help for our own feelings, such as guilt and aggression, so they do not vitiate our capacity to help.

In the UK, perhaps more than other countries the deepening centralisation of decision making and control of health care remains both disruptive and distracting. Public figures can work to their own agendas, often at cross purposes to the health needs of their populations. For health and social care organisations, the challenge is of sustaining what has been exemplary in this period, such as innovation in care, collaboration and courage in working across boundaries. This has required leadership at all levels, which is very separate from command and control that remains often the hallmark measures to deal with crisis. I have lost count of the numerous asks for pointless information from various sources and edicts to do whatever was the received wisdom of the day, which have added to the burden of colleagues trying to continue to deliver a service.

For the Trust, the challenge is growing what is special in our history, in delivering services over the past 100 years that have positively altered the societal view about marginalised service users, and increased knowledge and appreciation of their needs. By being active advocates of estranged and peripheral service user groups, we help promote an appreciation of societal wellbeing and the importance of addressing ill health in all its forms. Our strength is in our non pathologising stance, which often prevents a rush to intervene in unhelpful ways; and through our community interventions promoted safety and enriched lives, including by preventing hospitalisations during this period.

The pandemic has provided clear evidence of the indisputable connections between physical and mental health. It has also focussed our attention on the need to engage wider societal responses for the success of health measures aimed at the continuation of wellbeing. There are questions that need far greater exploration and effort to find resolution, such as who does the wealth of society serve, what is the meaning of economic growth if a section of a population suffers or dies and are we truly out of the pandemic if the social determinants of worse mortality are left unaddressed?

Finally, despite all the evidence of disproportionate impact on particular groups in society, there is a risk that we swing back to business as usual, with the usual hierarchies and privileges that caused the pandemic to wreck such havoc on our most vulnerable populations. In the coming period our challenge, as individuals and a health care system remains to hold onto our capacity to care for all in our communities who need our attention. We can help create oxygen for all to breathe more freely, by actively pushing back against conditions that promote neglect or that allow cruelty and everyday sadism to become dominant.

Disclosure statement

The main themes in the article were previously presented by the author at a Trust event.

References

Bandyopadhyay, S., Baticulon, R. E., Kadhum, M., Alser, M., Ojuka, D. K., Badereddin, Y., Kamath, A., Parepalli, S. A., Brown, G., Iharchane, S., Gandino, S., Markovic-Obiago, Z., Scott, S., Manirambona, E., Machhada, A., Aggarwal, A., Benazaize, L., Ibrahim, M., Kim, D., … Khundkar, R. (2020). Infection and mortality of healthcare workers worldwide from COVID-19: A systematic review. *BMJ Global Health Journal*, *5*(12), e003097. https://doi.org/10.1136/bmjgh-2020-003097

Benvenuto, S. (2016). *What are perversions?* Karnac books.

Dyer O. (2021). Covid-19: Study claims real global deaths are twice official figures. *BMJ*, *373*, n1188. https://doi.org/10.1136/bmj.n1188

Ellis, H. (1898–1928). Love and pain. In *Studies in the Psychology of Sex. Vols. 1–7*. F. Davis. [Revised edition in 4 volume published 1936, Random House.]

Fonagy, P. (1999). Male perpetrators of violence against women: An attachment theory perspective. *Journal of Applied Psychoanalytic Studies*, *1*, 7–27. https://doi.org/10.1023/A:1023074023087

Freiden, T. (2021, January 1). Which countries have responded best to Covid-19? *The Wall Street Journal*. https://www.wsj.com/articles/which-countries-have-responded-best-to-covid-19-11609516800?page=1

Glasser, M. (1988). Psychodynamic aspects of paedophilia. *Psychoanalytic Psychotherapy*, *3* (2), 121–135. https://doi.org/10.1080/02668738700700111

Gov.uk. (2021). https://coronavirus.data.gov.uk/details/deaths?areaType=overview&areaName=United%20Kingdom

Halliday, S. (2001). Death and miasma in Victorian London: An obstinate belief. *BMJ*, *323*(7327), 1469–1471. https://doi.org10.1136/bmj.323.7327.1469

Hegarty, S. (2020, February 6). *The Chinese doctor who tried to warn others about coronavirus*. BBC News. https://www.bbc.co.uk/news/world-asia-china-51364382.

Hutchinson, B. (2020 December 31). *Hospital CEO's response to Black doctor's COVID-19 death prompts backlash*. ABC news, coronavirus health and science. https://abcnews.go.com/US/hospitalceos-response-black-doctors-covid-19-death/story?id=74971005

Kirby, T. (2020). Evidence mounts on the disproportionate effect of COVID-19 on ethnic minorities. *The Lancet Respiratory Medicine*, *8*(6), 547–548. https://doi.org/10.1016/S2213-2600(20)30228-9

Klein, M. (1946). Notes on some schizoid mechanisms. *The International Journal of Psychoanalysis*, *27*(Pt 3–4), 99–110.

Klein, M. (1997). *Envy and gratitude: And other works, 1946-1963*. Random House. https://icd.who.int/browse11/l-m/en#/http://id.who.int/icd/entity/1890228613

Meere, M., & Egan, V. (2017). Everyday sadism, the dark train, personality and disgust sensitivity. *Personality and Individual Differences*, *112*, 157–161. https://doi.org/10.1016/j.paid.2017.02.056

Meloy, J., & Gacono, C. (1998). The internal world of the psychopath. In T. Millon, E. Simonsen, M. Birket-Smith, & R. D. Davis (Eds.), *Psychopathy: Antisocial, criminal, and violent behavior* (pp. 95–109). Guilford Press. https://www.researchgate.net/publication/287584013_The_internal_world_of_the_psychopath

Meloy, J. R. & Shiva, J. (2007). A psychoanalytic view of the psychopath. In A. Felthous, & H. Saß (Eds.), *The international handbook of psychopathic disorders and the law*. John Wiley & Sons, Ltd.

O'Meara, A., & Hammond, S. (2016). The sadistic impulse and relating to others. In J. Birtchnell, M. Newberry, & A. Kalaitzaki (Eds.), *Relating theory—Clinical and forensic applications* (pp. 277–291). Palgrave Macmillan. https://doi.org/10.1057/978-1-137-50459-3_21).

Platt, L., & Warwick, R. (2020) *Are some ethnic groups more vulnerable to COVID-19 than others?* IFS Deaton Review. https://ifs.org.uk/inequality/chapter/are-some-ethnic-groups-morevulnerable-to-covid-19-than-others/

World Health Organization (WHO). (2019). ICD-11 for mortality and morbidity statistics. Version: 2019. Retrieved August 20, 2019, from https://icd.who.int/browse11/l-m/en

Under fire in the consulting room

Carine Minne

A slow match is a very slow-burning fuse presenting only a small glowing tip whereas a quick match is one, which once ignited, burns at top speed. In this paper, I will present a number of clinical vignettes to illustrate situations when the therapist realised there was a sudden unexpected rise in 'temperature' of a patient's mind and why this may have occurred. A fuse was lit but was it a slow or a quick one? I will relate this ignition to the possibility of premature interpretations, or a failure to notice how anxious the patient was in the presence of the terrifying object-therapist and also, patients' unexpected responses to external interferences during a session. Descriptions of how these situations unfolded during sessions are given, and how, upon reflection, these could have been diffused differently. The emphasis will be on how best to maintain a psychoanalytic stance but also how to clinically judge when a session must be terminated in order to protect patient and therapist from exploding 'bombs' inadvertently ignited by patient or therapist. The importance of supervision and consultation with colleagues will be stressed.

It was a pleasure and honour to have been asked to come and present in celebration of the Tavistock and Portman's 100th anniversary thanks to Julian Stern, Ghazal Tipu and others behind the scenes for making it possible to transmit this Scientific Meeting using technology during these extraordinary and worrying pandemic times. I'd also like to thank Francesca Hume for agreeing to have chaired the zoom meeting.

I refer in the paper to clinical material about patients, some currently in treatment, and confidentiality is always a priority because without this, we cannot have patients in psychotherapy. I am grateful to my patients for agreeing to have extracts from their treatments used anonymously.

Needless to say, this pandemic has led us to making all kinds of adaptations to our ways of working, including the meeting where I originally presented this paper, that had to be held by zoom. I include a recent incident, which arose with a patient by phone shortly before the talk, where I did indeed feel under fire, as most certainly did the poor patient. I even had my first experience of a psychotherapy session whilst wearing Personal Protective Equipment (PPE) in the hospital I work in.

My intention is to present psychoanalytical work which did not run smoothly, or unexpected things came up and were dealt with in vivo, on the spot – but supervision and reflective practice afterwards would enable a forensic examination of the moment by moment happening, whether it was emotional, verbal or physical or all of the above.

I have referred in my abstract to fuses – these can be slow matches, when a glowing tip slowly ignites and there is a possibility of diffusing or halting the process, or quick matches, when, once ignited, burn at top speed. I will illustrate both types, some when the patients' mind had a slow rise in temperature and others when the rise in temperature was sudden. In all of these vignettes, I had to ask myself afterwards, what had I missed? What had I interpreted too soon? What was the patient needing to get rid of at that moment? Did I diffuse appropriately? Regular clinical supervision of these situations after they had occurred was always essential.

The Portman Clinic (Tavistock and Portman NHS Foundation Trust) is an out-patient psychotherapy clinic in London for adults, children and adolescents, young people and couples who are troubled or affected by violence and/or sexualized behaviours, legal or illegal. The patients at the Portman Clinic and in high security psychiatric hospitals are often people who have suffered unimaginable traumas in earlier lives by people responsible for their care. They cannot take for granted, like many of us might, that they will be reasonably treated. The tabloid press reports, and their experiences in prisons and other settings, confirm their familiar and worst suspicions; that they will be and deserve to be badly treated.

First, I describe a patient where the ignited fuse, a slow match, suddenly transformed into a quick match and the bomb very nearly did go off in the consulting room. I need to warn you that this man suffered from a life-threatening sexual perversion and that some of the details are appalling – the reason for presenting his case is not to cause distress, disgust or excitement but rather, to show just how much suffering there can be in patients caught up compulsively needing to act out an earlier undigested or unworked through trauma.

Mr. X first attended the Portman Clinic several years ago with what he described as 'a nervous breakdown'. His mother had died over a year earlier and, after a period of becoming physically unwell and having to live on sickness benefit, he immersed himself even more than before in dangerous sado-masochistic practices including beatings, bondage, partial asphyxiations, hangings, inserting various objects in his rectum, covering himself in faeces and at times, eating his own and other's faeces. He would then stop these practices completely for a few weeks at a time in an attempt to order his life again, only to succumb to the compulsion again. His life had fluctuated in this manner since his twenties but his perverse activities had increased in severity and frequency following the death of his mother. He wanted to find a balance between his extremes of living as (in his own words) 'totally bad or totally good'. He also desperately wanted to be able to work again.

At his assessment he presented as a pale, thin man, shabbily dressed, who walked slowly with a limp and who looked older than his age. At this time he was in his thirties. He seemed quite open and friendly and smelled of faeces. I knew straight away that my responses and countertransferences were likely to be very hard to manage. Hale (2020) has written about what he refers to as the autonomic countertransference, a concept that takes the concepts of projection and projective identification into the realm of reactions which can be provoked by certain psychopathological processes 'received' by a psychotherapist from a patient. The autonomic nervous system is a neural control system that acts largely unconsciously and regulates bodily functions and is the main system that leads to fight or flight responses. It is part of the peripheral nervous system that supplies smooth muscles including the digestive tract and glands and has sympathetic and parasympathetic branches, which respectively and generally, activate or inhibit physiological responses. As described by Hale (2020), one of these psychopathological processes, perverse sexuality can provoke a parasympathetic response within the psychotherapist's autonomic nervous system, that can lead to experiencing nausea. This response is in contrast to being exposed to violence, which provokes a sympathetic response, and fight or flight. It was understandable therefore why I was often left feeling nauseated during sessions with this patient. However, at those moments when a fuse became ignited, the countertransference was experienced via the sympathetic part of the autonomic nervous system, evoking a fight or flight reaction.

The patient did not say much about his family at the assessment but during treatment the following information came up. Mr X was the eldest of four children by his parent's marriage which was acrimonious. He described his father as physically very strong and a severe man who was never affectionate, who worked long hours in a factory, and who was not around much when they were children. He left home when Mr X was ten years old. He moved to Australia where he remarried and became a successful businessman. Mr X's mother, a housewife, was described by him as hysterical, violent and unpredictable. She started to beat the children more regularly after her husband left home, particularly focusing on Mr X. At times she would lock him in a cupboard for several hours or she would attempt to smother him with a pillow. The most lasting trauma sustained by him as a young child was a result of being hanged by her over the balcony of the 14th floor flat they lived in and later, I will illustrate how the impact of this continued to affect him. Diarrhoea from terror emerged from his bottom as he was held over the balcony upside down and reached his lips. This was not his first taste of faeces because, during the long course of our work together, we discovered that his mother used to smother him as a baby with his dirty nappy.

I will now present a session moment where Mr X nearly lost control when he briefly entered a psychotic phase and an avalanche of perverse fantasies arose as a desperate attempt on his part to try to contain his anxiety. He dragged up the stairs, taking much longer than usual to get to the room, looked very pale and miserable and told me he had been to the HIV information centre. He had to fill in a form and was told by the woman there to put down his symptoms at their worst (I thought he was already showing me his worst but I was wrong). He spoke about a sudden realization of how severely ill he really was.

He started staring at me intensely. He spoke to me about his confusion regarding being ill, asking himself was he really ill or did he put on being ill? He had told that woman at the HIV centre not to phone me and was very sorry that she probably had. He had tried to explain to her the nature of therapy and that she should not ask me for information about him but 'she said she knew best'. Suddenly, the voice of my colleague across the landing outside the consulting room then became audible and he described feeling irritated by her voice, reminding me that the same thing had happened the previous week. He wished she would shut up! He then spoke to me about masochistic practices and how he had always been the worst one, the most severe, that he felt at his worst right now and this all started a month ago when he had (once more) given up the sex practices and thrown away his equipment. I had said something to him the previous week which had affected him. He felt I had provoked him, that I was leading him on, and he had perceived me as having said 'say whatever is on your mind, your anxiety is only that I might crumble'. This had excited him a lot. He was still staring at me intensely and I was feeling very uncomfortable. He later said he had begun to have fantasies about me and had masturbated to these. His breathing had become very rapid in the session and he went on to say that he wanted to tell me the details but found this too difficult. Just the mere remembering aroused him. By this stage, he had started rocking backwards and forwards and was intensely staring at me. He wondered out loud what would happen if he just came right over and did it 'like put my cock in your mouth'. He was staring with his lips turned down, scowling, eyes wide, rocking and with a noticeable erection. I felt extremely anxious, trapped (to respond in any way could excite him even further) and I was worried something was just about to get out of control. I grappled with my thoughts and said to him that it sounded like it was me and my mouth he wanted to shut up rather than the voice we could vaguely hear outside. He responded by saying 'Yeah, that would fucking shut you up'. He continued to look very excited and mumbled something about wanting to tell me the details but not being able to. I said 'I think you want me to see you at your worst, it makes you very anxious and, instead, you get sexually excited'. He took a deep breath and said 'now I want to lick your vagina' in a very aggressive tone. I said 'perhaps what you remember of last week's session is very important, that is, how you perceive I respond to you'. 'Yes!' he snarled and shouted 'what would happen if ... ?' at which point I thought he was about to come over to me. I sat up straight and said firmly in a loud voice 'You know that to tell me the things on your mind can be helpful for us in our understanding of you, to actually do it would bring the session to an end and we would have lost the possibility of helping you with it'. This thankfully did seem to diffuse the situation and he took deep sighs and his body slumped back into his chair and his actual erection disappeared.

After a pause, he recounted the previous 3 years of therapy and said how different it felt for him being with me now. Also, giving up all the sex stuff again had made him worse. The first two years, he had wanted to be a model patient for me to find him interesting, write him up maybe as a famous case, like one of Freud's case histories. He had wanted to show me that he knew it all. He realized now that he did not, that this was not the point in coming here and he did feel himself becoming a real patient and actually having therapy rather than playing the part. Thinking about all the shit stuff, the mess, the disgust afterwards, he must be out of his mind. I commented on how out of his mind he may have felt a few minutes ago. He said 'Yeah and now I feel back in my mind' at which point he burst into tears, sobbing for several minutes. He said 'It feels as if something is changing for the first time since I was 14 years old. I hope I can stick with it'. I said I thought he hoped I was sufficiently robust and could stick with it with him.

From this case, you can see that something went terribly wrong from the beginning of the session. I had noticed his different appearance, his slowness in arriving up the stairs but I had not taken this up with him – I had not addressed the retrospectively obvious slow match. When he spoke about having gone to get help from the woman regarding his HIV status and been told to fill it in stating his worst, I could have intervened then and said something to him about him feeling the need to show his worst in case speaking it did not convey this sufficiently well. This might have diffused things at that moment as he might have felt understood. Instead, I let him continue to try to describe his worst, which he could not do verbally and had to resort to a physical manifestation. The slow match became a quick match at the point of interruption by an external noise – a colleague speaking loudly in the corridor outside our room, which amplified his distress at being convinced the HIV advisor had spoken to me – another intrusion (she had not tried to contact me). On the background of life-threatening intrusions from a disturbed murderous mother, these actual intrusions by women became focused on me as a woman, dangerous, threatening, and which he felt he had to defend himself against in the only way he knew how to in his grown-up body, with his perversion – the self-preservative violence being sexualised, as described by Glasser (1998).

Glasser introduced the concept of the *core complex*, formulated as a universal early experience, where the baby suffers from feelings of abandonment or, the opposite, engulfment in its micro- and macro- experiences of its mother or main carer. Aggression is a central component of the core complex and one way of managing these feelings if they become intolerable is to attempt to 'control' the object is by sexualizing the aggression. If core complex anxieties are not sufficiently contained by the mother or carer, a habitual sexualizing of aggression towards significant others arises, which can lead to the development of a sexual perversion. Returning to Mr X, to put his cock in my mouth would be a sexualized aggression and would have certainly shut me up – possibly for good. I would also experience a version of what he had experienced – a suffocation – a reversal for him of an early repeated trauma. If there was more space, I would have elaborated on the relevance of the previous sessions in laying the ingredients for this bomb arising at that particular session.

Strangely enough, in all the years working in high security, I have only had to use the emergency buzzer twice for the nurses to come urgently to the room because a patient had 'exploded'. Twice it was with the same patient, a female. Once, early on in treatment, she suddenly got up and tried to throw her chair at me. I had made the error of a premature maternal transference interpretation and, given her experience of having had a 'perverse' mother as described by Welldon (1988), my use of the word mother linked to me was intolerable. Welldon has written about how, in contrast to men suffering from perversions, women use their entire bodies, or extensions of their bodies, which includes their babies, to express their suffering, meaning that their babies are also victims of their mother's perversion. This was a young woman, who was victim of her own disturbed mother and who subsequently killed her baby and I have often spoken about her in clinical meetings and presentations previously because she taught me so much. She received a conviction for infanticide. Psychoanalytically however, I think this killing could also be understood as a case of matricide and of suicide. I hope to show how this killing of the baby involved shifting identifications in the patient-mother, from being her disturbed self, to being identified with her own disturbed mother and being identified with the baby.

Ms B developed concerns about her baby soon after the birth. She was convinced that the baby was sick and called her Health Visitor and family doctor regularly but could never accept reassurance. When the baby was 9 weeks old, she again made contact saying that the baby had started manifesting facial tics like her own of such severity that the baby's breathing was affected. She and the baby were admitted to hospital for the baby to be monitored. Initially, the baby was found to be well but after two days, the baby's condition began to deteriorate for which no cause could be found. The baby became critically ill, was transferred to intensive care and died.

Ms B, manifestly distressed, went home with her mother. Soon after the baby's death and post-mortem, laboratory reports showed toxic levels in the baby's blood of the medication Ms B was on for her own facial tic disorder and confirming the cause of death. She was arrested and charged with murdering her baby. Her early weeks on remand were spent in a women's prison before she was transferred to a secure psychiatric unit because she became withdrawn and uncommunicative. Ms B eventually admitted having given the baby her medication, not to kill the baby but out of concern that the doctors and nurses were not looking after the baby properly. Retrospectively, it could be suggested that she projected her own bad experience of being mothered twice over, once into her own baby, by identifying with her mother and then again, by projective identification with the nurses and doctors, who became the bad parents for not noticing what was going on within the sick baby, herself, as well as the actual sick baby.

Ms B started twice-weekly psychoanalytical psychotherapy with me following her transfer to high security, where, as before in medium security, she became a 'model', compliant patient. During the early months of treatment with me, she presented as a distressed patient who spoke about what a dreadful thing she had done but this had a pseudo-feel to it. This way of presenting to me was gradually shown to her and interpreted as one way she had of avoiding feeling traumatized or victimized by her own disturbed state of mind at the time of her offences and now, in the room with me.

Later, she occasionally became more able to speak to me about what she did to her baby, how she crushed her tablets and secretly fed this to the baby, over and over again. At these moments, her real distress was very apparent. She described her preoccupation at the time with her belief that the baby was not being looked after properly by the nurses and doctors. I said to her, at these moments in her sessions, how she wished to be the baby that could be looked after properly. This was a highly ambivalent situation for this patient where she was faced with the problem that to be looked after properly negated her view of what proper looking after within her family structure meant, creating a sense of betraying her family if she followed the trend of her therapy. I had to be kept, therefore, as someone who was bound to harm her in some way and her history and offence were once more re-enacted.

The pathological mother-child dynamic present in this patient's mind could also be seen in her therapy when she took an overdose before a session and then appeared with glazed eyes and bilateral hand tremor. She denied several times that anything was the matter when her physical state was commented on, before becoming angry and shouting that there was no point in all this, she wanted to be with her baby, another reference to her suicidality. She kept me in a concerned state and, after considering the likelihood of her having taken an overdose, I told her that I thought she wanted me to be a good mother and guess what was the matter. This was followed by a long silence. I said I believed she would be relieved if I guessed. I then told her I thought she wanted me to know she had taken an overdose. If I did not notice this, she could congratulate herself that she was right, no one notices she is serious (about suicide). If I did notice, she would get something from me but it would feel spoilt because of how she got it. In this situation, the patient did finally admit to having taken an overdose, which had to be urgently dealt with, medically. Again, in this session, the offence is repeated, a baby, herself, is harmed, again with medication, but this time the baby is saved. Indeed, the 'being saved' actually led to a manic outburst of profuse thanks from the patient, diluting the seriousness of what had just happened and avoiding the experience of guilt that such a saving could provoke.

I had to reflect afterwards in supervision what could have been done better in such a session. Should I have immediately commented on her unwell physical appearance right at the start and said that it looked as if she'd taken an overdose and we should stop and get medical attention? If I had done this, would we have lost the opportunity to gain some understanding there and then of why she was doing what she did?

In March 2020, the global Covid pandemic finally led to lockdown of the whole of England, meaning that out-patient psychotherapy clinics, including the Portman Clinic, were closed. Psychotherapists everywhere had to rapidly adjust to alternate ways of maintaining regular contact with patients, including telephone or audio-visual computer sessions. Within 4 weeks of the lockdown starting, I got through by telephone to one of my female patients who had a history of violence some years back. I expected her, like most of the patients had, to just let me know they were OK and talk a bit about their situation in lock down. Instead she screamed down the phone and finally was able to convey that she had felt like killing her husband and had instead, locked him out in the garden. I could hear him shouting and their young child crying in the background. This was a family known to me since the birth of the child a few years ago. After finding a way of calming her down, I asked her to hand the phone to her husband through the kitchen window. I listened and spoke to him for about 15 minutes too – and was able to piece together with them both what the trigger had been for this acute relapse between them. I was also able to speak to the child, who told me 'I am happy you phoned because mummy and daddy have been fighting again and I couldn't get them to stop but I think you will'. The child had met me many times over the years since her babyhood so I was not a stranger to her and she also had therapy when she was younger with a colleague. I then talked to the woman again and together we made a highly structured written plan of how best for them to manage, including letting the man in, which occurred whilst I stayed on the phone. A plan was made for a further call later that day and this later call confirmed that the acute situation was diffused – but we all agreed it could of course arise again. The two adults said that having a planned structure helped and they had sellotaped it to their fridge so they knew what to do when the family/couple 'temperature' rises again. They also had other emergency phone services they could call out of hours when I was not available. I immediately contacted (with her knowledge) her local community mental health team so they were aware that their assistance may also be required and her medication might need to be reviewed sooner than in the planned three months later.

In terms of bombs in the consulting room, was this a slow match or a quick match? I think it was both – the tension of lockdown in a small flat together had risen over the previous few weeks and then, a quick match, or trigger, had ignited the big row.

All three vignettes, very different cases though they are, have a common theme. In each case, the patient suffered unimaginable and uncontained distress in babyhood. Mr X experienced a disturbed mother who either neglected him or was trying to kill him through suffocation. In terms of Glasser's core complex referred to earlier, he experienced what I can only call an extreme core complex as a baby, either utterly lost as if an astronaut floating away in space or literally suffocated. Both these extreme ends of the core complex spectrum will have led to him needing to develop extreme methods to survive. Disgusting as his sexualized aggressive behaviours were, seen in this context, one could consider these as astonishingly creative attempts by his mind to preserve his life. Ms B was also exposed to a mother who either neglected her or exposed her to paedophilic men, which she herself, the patient's mother, had experienced and who, sadly, was never offered help. The third vignette, the female patient 'seen' by telephone during a pandemic lockdown crisis, also had baby traumas. She was the last and unwanted child by her parents, her mother sending her as much as possible to be looked after by two older sisters who resented the task and she also experienced extended periods of neglect. Welldon (2012) has also emphasized the importance of exploring the trans-generational aspects of abuse and how these terrible cycles of abuse are 'transmitted'. Mr X made a decision very early in his young adulthood that he would never have children as he thought he could never trust himself to care for any child adequately. Ms B was most certainly part of a trans-generationally repeated abuse and what a tragedy that her baby daughter ended up being killed. The third patient was able to access help just in time so that her daughter did not suffer what she had suffered, although this child was still exposed to her parents' vulnerabilities, but at least with the knowledge and experience of there being other adults in her life to support the whole family.

Certain dangerous fuses at risk of igniting are those in the consulting rooms emanating from understandable organizational anxieties with their focus on bureaucratic manoeuvres and procedures designed to extinguish risk as they are designed to do and as first described by Menzies-Lythe (1959). Those 'fuses' most at risk of igniting are when clinicians do not access supervision, so essential in our clinical work. The importance of the third in such cases-and indeed in less extreme cases, cannot be over emphasised. I would have exposed my patients to a further betrayal if I had not accessed regular supervision and for this, I remain grateful not only to my patients from whom I learnt so much but also to my supervisors who taught me and provided containment at crucial times. For patients treated in in-patient settings, reflective practice for the whole clinical team is essential in order to provide some immunity to the high risk of all staff otherwise inadvertently acting out to what can be evoked or provoked by the patients' historical and current suffering. Without supervision, there can be no psychotherapy.

Disclosure statement

No potential conflict of interest was reported by the author(s).

References

Glasser, M. (1998). On violence: A preliminary communication. *International Journal of Psychoanalysis*, *79*, 887–902.

Hale, R. (2020). Autonomic counter-transference: The psychopathic mind and the institution. *The International Journal of Forensic Psychotherapy*, *2*(2), 101–112. https://doi.org/10.33212/ijfp.v2n2.2020.101

Menzies-Lythe, I. (1959). The functioning of social systems as a defence against anxiety. *Human Relations 13*, 95–121. https://doi.org/10.1177/001872676001300201

Welldon, E. V. (1988). *Mother, Madonna, Whore*. Free Association Books.

Welldon, E. V. (2012). Bodies across generations and cycles of abuse. In P. Mariotti (Ed.), *The maternal lineage. Identification,desire and transgenerational issues. The new library of psychoanalysis* (pp. 381–401). Routeledge.

The Fitzjohn's Unit

David Bell and Birgit Kleeberg

This article provides a description of the development and work of The Fitzjohn's Unit a specialist service, housed within the Adult Department of the Tavistock and Portman NHS Foundation Trust, providing psychoanalytic psychotherapy for patients suffering from the more complex/serious disorders many of them having been unwell for many decades. The paper describes the patients treated, the model of care and also aims to show how this work can illuminate more general consideration such as the nature of the psychoanalytic attitude and the relation of psychiatry to psychoanalysis

The Fitzjohn's Unit began life in 2000, evolving as part of the clinical services of the then Adult Department of the Tavistock and Portman NHS Foundation Trust and embedded within the department's psychoanalytic culture. It was started as an experimental project by David Taylor. David Bell became the lead consultant in 2002. Not long after that Edna O'Shaughnessy, a distinguished senior psychoanalyst, was invited to join the unit as its external supervisor. There had, for some time previously, been a broad recognition that a significant group of patients were particularly disadvantaged by the limitations of the generic treatment model of the Adult Department which offered once-weekly psychotherapy for one year. These individuals tended to suffer from more serious levels of pervasive and long-term disturbance and we recognised that, after a year's treatment, we had only just *begun* to make any significant contact with them and that, in some cases, ending the therapy then risked losing even the small gains we had made. It was therefore decided to develop a specialist unit that could address these patients in a more appropriate manner and over the following year or two we developed the model which has become the foundation of our work.

We created a specialised service where patients receive twice-weekly sessions of individual psychotherapy for two years with an experienced psychotherapist, followed by group psychotherapy for a further number of years. This model was adopted and adapted from one used at the Cassel Hospital, an inpatient therapeutic community for more disturbed patients, where both David Bell and Birgit Kleeberg had previously worked at different times.

In 2003, the UK Government published a document, *Personality disorder: no longer a diagnosis of exclusion*, highlighting the plight of patients with long-term disorders arising from profound character problems who were excluded from mental health services (on the grounds that they did not suffer from *illnesses*, as such). This proved to be strategically very useful in the development of the Fitzjohn's Unit, in that it provided incentives for other services to refer this group of patients to us.

While encouraging the referral of patients with features of personality disorder, we also attempt to retain a broader remit in terms of types of the patients we accept. Unlike most personality disorder services, we do not insist that our patients meet formal diagnostic criteria for personality disorder. Our broader inclusion criteria thus give us a unique place amongst other local services and this is increasingly appreciated by referrers and patients alike.

By representing the work of the unit, both internally within the Trust (to Board of the Trust, for example) and externally (by establishing links with the heads of other services), David Bell enabled us to provide better, longer-term care for our patients. Clinicians from other services within the Trust are encouraged to bring complex cases for discussion in the unit meeting. We are also approached to consult to mental health services from other trusts, such as inpatient teams struggling to manage a particularly difficult patient. Occasionally an invitation will be issued to the team to come to our unit meeting to present the situation that they are struggling with. The ensuing discussion then also provides a learning opportunity for all the members of our own unit.

Having worked in the unit from its inception, Birgit Kleeberg joined David Bell as co-manager in 2005. We have developed a model of sharing the responsibility of leading the unit between two people which has worked very well (it is the only clinical unit in the adult service that is managed in this way). This again leans on our experience at the Cassel Hospital, where we had learnt the value of a 'couple' – psychotherapist /primary nurse or consultant/senior nurse – working together to contain various levels of disturbance.

In addition to the unit meeting, there is another weekly meeting, the staff seminar led by Edna O'Shaughnessy,[1] who does not attend the unit meeting. This forum is restricted to those who have patients in treatment – it is not open to outside visitors. David Bell made a decision not to attend this seminar so that it could proceed unconstrained by the consideration of management issues. Highly valued by the staff group, the staff seminar provides a space to think together freely and creatively. An important feature of the seminar is that clinical work is presented and discussed in an open and trusting manner, centring on the material brought and taking care to eschew judgment of the therapist. There is a strong sense of communal responsibility and the expression 'we are all with you' has been adopted as a kind of wry mantra; it seems to capture and acknowledge *both* the reality of being on one's own with the patient *and* the solidarity provided by the group. This structure has enabled us to create and maintain strong staff morale, perhaps one of the most critical factors necessary for containing the high levels of disturbance created by the nature of this work.

The clinicians on the unit are all qualified, experienced psychotherapists, many of whom had their psychotherapy training in the Adult Department. A substantial number are psychiatrists and/or psychoanalysts whilst others have a background in in the humanities. We provide an advanced two-year clinical training for qualified psychotherapists who wish to learn about working with more disturbed patients. As honorary psychotherapists on the unit, they are each assigned a patient under supervision and are also provided with a theoretical course. They contribute greatly to the life of the unit. The diversity of the staff group, who originate from different countries, and are from various intellectual and professional backgrounds and schools of thought within psychoanalysis, makes it a rich and rewarding environment to work in.

How people become our patients

Referrals to the unit come from a number of sources, regularly from GPs and psychiatrists based in local mental health, but also from psychology, Improving Access to Psychological Therapies (IAPT), and student counselling services. The large majority of patients referred proceed to assessment. However, the term assessment is perhaps not quite right, as it might suggest a kind of examination, a test to be passed or failed. When conducting our assessments, we are, in fact, not looking to the patients to prove themselves in any way as 'suitable'. Our default position is that the patient can be helped unless there are very good reasons which make it unwise to proceed, for example, if there is an unacceptably high risk of deeper engagement. The psychoanalytic assessment consultation provides the foundation on which all subsequent engagement is built.

One might expect that someone's availability for understanding, their capacity to be interested in their own mind, requires the person to be relatively less disturbed, but we have found there is no simple relation between level of disturbance and psychotherapeutic availability. It is not unusual to find that very disturbed patients, including some who would be classed as psychotic, respond well to attempts to understand them and go on to make good use of psychotherapy. (For a more detailed account of our approach to assessments, see Bell & Kleeberg, 2013.)

Inevitably, because of limitations on our resources, patients have to wait – often for many months – before they can begin psychotherapy. Some patients find this too difficult and drop off the waiting list. This was, we thought, partly a result of having been invited into the intimate and disturbing contact of the assessment, but then feeling left to manage on their own. As a result of an audit which revealed this problem we decided to ensure that all patients on the waiting list need to continue to be reviewed by the assessor, at varying intervals whilst on the waiting list, usually every four to six weeks. This enables a continuing containment which helps them manage and so sustain their engagement.

As is perhaps already clear, the patients are not only disturbed but also disturbing. We have found it helpful to insist that no individual clinician in the unit take full or exclusive responsibility for any patient. When difficulties threaten to lead to a breakdown in the relationship between patient and therapist, the assessor becomes a case manager who can step in to manage the situation and help the patient to remain in therapy.

This separation of responsibilities between the psychotherapist and the person who helps to manage crises makes for a much better structure and so, wherever possible, we try to ensure that the psychotherapist offering treatment is never the same person who was the assessor.

The assessor also carries out the review which usually takes place a few months after a patient has completed their individual psychotherapy. This meeting aims to help them reflect upon what has been achieved and whether or not they are interested in entering the second phase of the treatment programme, group psychotherapy. The conclusion of the group treatment marks another juncture where they might again touch base with the assessor. Although inevitably straining our limited resources, this structure enables us to provide a continuity of care which is an essential part of treatment approach.

Many of our patients are concurrently being managed by local mental health services, something we actively encourage, particularly as, given we are not an emergency service, we cannot provide availability in an acute crisis. It is, of course, important to maintain close liaison with these services, while at the same time protecting the psychotherapy itself from potentially damaging intrusions. Again, the person responsible for this kind of liaison is not the psychotherapist, but the assessor or, on occasion, another therapist on the unit. Whenever the patient is discussed at a unit meeting, we ensure that both the psychotherapist and the case manager are present. Thus the boundary between the two functions can perhaps best be described as a kind of 'semi-permeable membrane'.

A more detailed look at who our patients are

An audit of cases referred to the Unit over a two-year period (2011–2013) showed that the average age of patients was forty years and 77% of them were female. The picture that emerged was of a patient group with longstanding serious difficulties, usually dating from childhood or adolescence (69%). The majority report having had problems within themselves, in their relationships with others for as long as they can remember and many have found social interaction unmanageably exhausting. Some feel they lose their sense of self when with others and yet on their own they feel very alone and empty. Many say they don't want to be alive, that they are unable to move forward and feel stuck forever in a 'living hell'.

A significant number of our patients have been given multiple diagnoses over the years. Diagnoses of discrete disorders such as recurrent depressive disorder or bipolar disorder is common, but these labels do no justice to the complexity and depth of their difficulties. This depression is not really recurrent, it is on-going and life-long – it might more accurately be described as a depressive personality disorder with occasional manic episodes. Others fulfil the diagnostic criteria for bipolar disorder but again, a large proportion of our patients have a history of emotional and physical childhood abuse or of other major traumas; suicidality and self-harm are common. The damage they inflict on themselves can take many different forms, such as restriction of food, binging and vomiting, cutting and burning themselves, overdosing on pain killers, and severe bouts of drinking. Some will have had periods of compulsory hospitalisation during manic or depressive episodes.

The majority of patients treated on the unit will have been unable to sustain employment for many years, sometimes despite good academic achievements. Others manage to hold down jobs but become troubled when they are promoted to positions which bring new stresses, the most difficult change often being one that requires the patient to deal more directly with greater numbers of people. A few manage quite demanding jobs by detaching themselves from their disturbance and living their lives in a cut-off/dissociated state. In such cases, when the psychotherapy progresses, defences can temporarily break down and work colleagues then become more aware of the patients' difficulties. This, of course, needs careful managing.

Our patients have usually had many previous therapeutic interventions – including medication, other forms of psychotherapy, and psychiatric admissions – before they are referred to our service. This high proportion of failed previous attempts at treatment indicates a group of people who, because of the toxic transferences they form, find it difficult to establish a constructive relationship with the appropriate professionals. In some cases, these difficulties have been expressed in the form of a formal complaint against their local service. This is a special group where the outcome is very difficult to predict: some are able to work through the complaint and engage in a therapeutic process, while for others history unfortunately repeats itself. However, even in these situations – that is, where a complaint is made against our service – we try to continue to work with the patient to try to understand the nature of the complaint and the psychic reasons for making it. In some cases, this has led to a good therapeutic outcome.

The audit found that the most common ICD 10 diagnoses were recurrent depression (F33), a specific personality disorder (F60), and bipolar affective disorder (F31). Forty-three per cent of the cohort presented with some form of diagnosable personality disorder (the largest group being borderline), 63% with serious affective disorder. The most common comorbidities were between these two diagnoses.

Assessment reports highlighted the presence of suicidality in 40% of the sample; post-traumatic stress disorder (PTSD), dissociation, a history of abuse, or severe trauma appeared in 46%; personality disorder, including paranoid traits, were detected in a third; 20% manifested self-destructiveness, self-hatred, and the risk of harmful behaviour to the self. In terms of psychoanalytic formulation, the most commonly observed qualities were suppressed rage, self-hatred, narcissism and grandiosity, and dissociation. In half of cases, there was explicit mention of physical health problems, with a quarter having physical symptoms possibly related to mental health disorders, including eating disorders; 23% presented with what were apparently psychosomatic disorders. The frequency of comments relating to previous failed attempts at treatment (57%) indicates a population that finds it very difficult to establish a constructive relationship to sources of help or is particularly sensitive to inadequacies in the care provided. Just over half the sample was unemployed.

Just over half of referred patients were offered treatment; of these, a quarter were categorised as 'declining treatment'.

This is a patient group who are heavily predisposed to developing serious psychological disorders, through a combination of endowment /predisposition and disturbing experiences early in life. It is impossible, to disentangle one from the other. Whatever their origins, because these early developmental processes have not been worked through successfully, they continue to dominate the lives of these patients, leaving them limited in their emotional capacity and vulnerable to breakdown.

Inevitably, the frightening and persecuting inner objects are transferred into the relationship with the psychotherapist, who may thus have to bear long periods of being experienced in a very negative manner. The therapist's capacity to endure this requires considerable experience and can be of the utmost importance for the patient's welfare. In this way, tormenting relationships can be relived and worked with in their present manifestation and gradually, over time, be modified.

At the same time, patients also develop a capacity to contain their own disturbing states of mind and this, in turn, creates a greater self-awareness and self-acceptance, and a capacity to see others as they really are. These psychological developments can bring about reparative wishes and an increased ability to consider another person not only as an object in their world, but as a subject with their own history and experience. This provides a basis for an improved, more benign interpersonal relating and thus a break with the previous vicious circle of repetition.

Our aims are modest. We do not expect very ill patients to emerge from therapy in a radically altered state. Indeed, it is often a major achievement – for the psychotherapist as well as the patient – to throw off the tyrannical idea that the patient must recover. Even those who are unable to change very much can find the experience of being understood and accepted as both profound and immensely valuable. Some patients may realise that they will always be prone to disturbance, but they may nonetheless feel that something important has been achieved (particularly the experience of being understood).

Psychoanalysis and psychiatry

Psychoanalysis and psychiatry occupy conceptual domains that do not map onto each other precisely, are not symmetrical. Psychiatric theory and practice are informed by a large number of conceptually distinct paradigms. Some of these paradigms can live more or less happily alongside each other whilst others are in direct contradiction; some are entirely consistent with a psychoanalytic perspective, but others are, to varying degrees, opposed to the whole approach that psychoanalysis represents. If one thinks, for example, of the situation where a patient requires medication, much may depend upon the context within which it is given. Where this context emphasises an understanding of the psychological development of the illness and its meaning within current personal and social circumstances, there is no contradiction with psychoanalysis. But where the illness is understood as a purely *biological* phenomenon, distinct from the person in which it manifests itself, where the person is viewed as a passive recipient of a pathological process (an object of this process, not a subject), then the contradiction with a psychoanalytic perspective is clear.[2]

The Fitzjohn's Unit started life in a psychiatric context very different, if not categorically different, from the present one. That is, where we are now bears some relation to where we were then, but there has been an evolution of sorts – regrettably, not a developmental one. Twenty years ago, there was much more general acceptance that psychiatric theory and practice are necessarily informed by a large number of conceptually distinct paradigms, as touched upon above. That is, differing models of mental illness, though representing fundamentally different attitudes to mental suffering, had to cohabit and this gave breadth and richness to psychiatry. A proper understanding of psychiatric disorder involved considering the individual in relation to his current social context and his psychological past, as well as to his existence as a biological being. Psychiatric training would involve acquiring a certain familiarity with these competing paradigms, thus encouraging a capacity to live with ambiguity, an essential quality for a psychiatrist. In our current world, this multifaceted richness is in danger of being completely lost as one particular attitude to psychiatric illness is in danger of achieving hegemony.

When the unit began, the service was unusual but not strikingly at odds with the general psychiatric context. Many referrers recognised that some kinds of psychological disturbance require long-term treatment and valued the kind of thinking, liaison, and continuity of care that we were able to offer. However, our service has increasingly come to be at odds with other mental health care provision as services have been reduced, curtailed, and fragmented in response to cost-cutting measures, performance targets, and financial pressures. As a result, psychiatric liaison has become very difficult and sometimes impossible in a context where patients can only be provided with the required care if there is a crisis – a crisis which might have been averted if the previously existing structures of care had not been dismantled.

The general recognition that many kinds of psychological disturbance require long-term treatment and continuity of care has been replaced by an attitude of short-term-ism, with catastrophic consequences. For example, until recently, day hospitals provided a non-toxic environment where patients could gradually develop interpersonal skills and receive emotional support in a structured context; this required stays of many months, often more than a year. However, these centres have been re-designated as 'recovery centres'. The implication and expectation is that in a quite limited amount of time, measured in weeks, patients can recover from years of mental illness and return to ordinary living. This not only bears no relation to the reality of these patients' difficulties, but also creates a tyranny for the staff. The patients are *supposed* to recover, and there are performance targets against which this will be judged. If they do not recover, the implied conclusion is that the service or staff have failed.

What is missing here is any recognition that a great deal of the care of those with enduring mental illness has more to do with damage limitation and providing forms of support and care, skills which are much less valued today. Day hospitals were often staffed by teams established over many years and composed of individuals with high levels of skill. The de-skilling process, driven by financial pressures, has resulted in patients being often looked after by well-intentioned individuals who have virtually no experience of working with the mentally ill.

By perverse logic, some of these changes in health care are presented as providing the patient with more freedom of choice. In reality, the 'choice agenda' serves to make people believe they have more freedom in order to mask the fact that they have less. Patients cannot choose a service that has been closed.

Patients with these longer-term difficulties need to have continuing contact with the psychiatric teams that had provided their care in the past and would do so in the future. This on-going contact provides a vital consistency of care. Many have told us what a relief it is to have this kind of continuity, and so are not required to keep repeating their story to each new service or practitioner and, perhaps most importantly, they feel a sense of containment from the knowledge that that those looking after them now have previously known them at their worst. Here, real understanding that patients are sometimes damaged by institutionalisation has been twisted into a perverse justification for not providing the services they can depend upon.

Psychiatric liaison, which remains an important part of our work on the Fitzjohn's Unit has become increasingly difficult to achieve in a context where services have been so radically cut and fragmented. Maintaining and indeed continuously expanding the unit in this changed climate has, we believe, been a very considerable achievement.

Nomothetic and ideographic levels of description

The foregoing can be further elucidated by considering what is perhaps one of the most important tensions in the practice of psychiatry and within psychology in general, namely between the 'nomothetic' and 'ideographic' levels of description. The nomothetic seeks to group together objects that are similar into a categories (for example vegetables, forms of transport, infectious diseases), whereas the ideographic aims to capture the unique qualities of an individual case. When we characterise someone as depressed or as suffering from a psychosis, we are using the nomothetic level of description and we hope that classifying phenomena in this manner will be helpful in various ways, such as suggesting the likely course of the illness, prognosis, treatment, and so on. Or, when we suggest that a particular kind of mental state tends to be associated with specific forms of transference, we again give emphasis to the nomothetic characteristics they share. The ideographic, on the other hand, explores the individual, sometimes unique, qualities of any object. Clearly, there must be both levels of description for rational discourse to take place.

Over time, however – and with increasing momentum – this tension is being lost as our discipline is overtaken by the hegemony of classifications and diagnostic labels. Patients are now shoe-horned into discrete categories and mental illness 'clusters' that have pre-prescribed packages of care and prices attached (e.g., Lee et al., 2011), thus serving the needs of a market-oriented system and of the insurance and pharmaceutical industries.

This commodification of mental suffering pushes mental health workers to treat patients not as individuals, but as the carriers of diagnostic categories. This has resulted in profound feelings of alienation and loss of morale among mental health workers, a crucial element in healthcare and one which is largely absent from health policy, which tends to focus on 'skill mixes' rather than people.

The psychoanalytic approach, by contrast, requires the sustaining of this tension between the general and the particular, always preserving an emphasis on the ideographic, whether at the level of the individual person or in the detailed discussion of a particular session. This approach thus finds itself increasingly at odds with the mental health system and so its place has been reduced to a fraction of what it once was. We are not saying that the impoverishment of psychiatric services is a direct result of the reduced presence of psychoanalysis, as such. It is due, rather, to the loss of the kind of *psychiatric weltanschauung* in which this kind of thinking has a natural place.

The psychoanalytic attitude

Implicit in much of the above is the distinctiveness of the psychoanalytic approach, which characterises a central core of the Tavistock tradition and underpins all the work of the unit. It might now be helpful to examine in more detail some core elements of the psychoanalytic attitude.

Mrs A, a woman in her forties, was referred for an assessment for psychotherapy. She had suffered from chronic depression for over ten years and had already undergone a raft of treatments to no avail. When invited to tell me of her difficulties at the beginning of the consultation she gave me a detailed, and in many ways, very competent account of the illness, much of which consisted of going through a list of symptoms, how long she had had them, how her life was affected, etc. The atmosphere, however, was one of utter lifelessness: she talked only of her symptoms and not of herself and it felt as if she was handing her 'ill self' over to me, positioning herself as a passive object. I pointed this out to her, saying that she appeared to be wanting to give me a list of all the things that assailed her, to hand them over to me for diagnosis and recommendation for treatment, without having to participate in this process at all. Suddenly there was a change in the atmosphere. She started weeping and said, 'I don't think I have ever participated in anything in my life'. An important move had taken place: she had become much more alive and, paradoxically, by talking of not participating, the patient was now participating in the interview in a way that was very real, but also quite disturbing to her.

This brief vignette serves to characterise a number of features that are essential to the psychoanalytic attitude: an individual's suffering cannot be properly characterised as an 'illness', for it is always the expression of a whole personality and it is only through an engagement that foregrounds the relationship in the consulting room that the psychopathology can be grasped as a *dynamic* structure that enables one to form an adequate assessment of the patient's difficulties and what they are seeking, at both a conscious and less conscious level.

The term psychoanalysis covers a wide conceptual range but can be encompassed within the following broad categories: a body of knowledge about the mind, a research method, and a way of treating mental disorder. It is useful to keep this broad frame of reference in mind because, in discussions of psychoanalysis in the context of psychiatry, it is easy to slip into thinking of it solely as a form of treatment for individual patients. This is an important misunderstanding, for it is as a direct consequence of its range that psychoanalysis has had so much to contribute to the understanding and treatment of mental illness.

Normality and abnormality

Psychoanalysis does not investigate the human condition from the perspective of 'normality'; for all psychoanalysts since Freud, this has been a convenient fiction. The relation of the abnormal to the normal in psychoanalysis is more complex and more problematic. Careful study of the abnormal reveals what the normal hides, shows what is immanent in it. To paraphrase Freud, the neurotic speaks loudly about what the rest of us keep secret. It was his appreciation of what was revealed in delusions of being observed – an abnormal phenomenon – that led Freud to appreciate the depth and archaic qualities of the normal primitive superego. Even within the most ordinary and most disregarded aspects of mental life (such as slips and symptoms), Freud finds profound and sublime aspects of the human struggle.

In 'Obsessive actions and religious practices', Freud (1907) showed the parallel between the strange, private ceremonials and rituals of the obsessional neurotic and certain religious practices. Both centre on the need to keep separate good and bad, the sacred and the profane. Both have intense feelings of guilt, and ways of dealing with it, as central to their content. The difference is that obsessional rituals are idiosyncratic to the individual, whereas religious ceremonials are collective and stereotyped. Freud goes on to say (referring to the difference between neurotic symptoms and the achievements of culture): 'The divergence resolves itself ultimately into the fact that the neuroses are asocial structures; they endeavour to achieve by private means what is effected in society by collective effort' (Freud, 1907, p. 73). This demonstration of the continuities between the apparently bizarre or abnormal and so-called normality, the insight that the achievements of human culture and the manifestations of human neurosis have more in common than our narcissism would like to regard as acceptable, is typical of Freud's thought.

Freud's attitude to religion is symmetrical to his attitude to psychiatric disorder. He showed considerable respect for the contradictory nature of both of these human creations: they are at one and the same time expressions of human problems *and* of our attempts to resolve them; they display what is highest and what is lowest in our nature. Thus, psychoanalysis humanises our attitude to mental illness, serving as a useful brake on those culturally endorsed projective systems that seek to view those suffering from mental illness as fundamentally 'other', not like ourselves.

Ms T formed a precipitately idealised relationship with her psychotherapist whom she saw as different from the psychiatrists she had seen; they were 'not interested in me but only in their theories'. In one session, the therapist made a mistake as to the age of her son. Suddenly the atmosphere changed, as she turned on him with scorn and contempt, saying that now she could see he was no different from anyone else; he obviously had never been listening to her at all. The atmosphere was now one of utter hopelessness. A few weeks later, she recounted that as a child she would escape from a very disturbing situation at home by 'holing up' in some caves nearby and painting over all the cracks in the cave with 'magic paint' in order to 'stop the monsters getting in'.

One might say that she had, in the early phase of her therapy, used the magic paint of idealisation to create for herself a kind of personal sacred space in the treatment – the cave of her childhood – where she could feel safe. The therapist's mistake, however, opened a crack in the idealisation and now all the monsters could get in, as her attack on the therapist had made manifest.

And now a very different situation:

When the emergency team visited Mrs X, a known patient with a history of psychotic illness, they found her in a terrified state. She had covered all the windows and doors with Sellotape. This was, she explained, to prevent the evil rays getting into her flat.

These two examples, one of a more neurotic situation and the other more clearly psychotic, serve to show how, despite the gross differences in mental state of the two patients, the content of their preoccupations is very similar. Each patient worked to create an idealised retreat, a kind of personal religion, where they could find protection from destructive forces. In both cases, the destructive forces are felt to exist in the external world (the fantasied monsters in Ms T's case, the evil rays in Mrs X's case). The content of the preoccupations is thus similar for both patients but the *form* it takes is quite distinct.

Historical continuity – a developmental perspective

An important related feature of psychoanalytic explanation lies in its commitment to historical continuity. Freud's *Three Essays on Sexuality* (Freud, 1905) provided not only a model of sexual development and an understanding of the sexual perversions, but introduced a method of *understanding disorder in terms of development*. Disorder makes manifest certain aspects of mental life which, at a different developmental phase (for example, in early childhood) might well have been normal. Although we never completely lose earlier ways of functioning, when these more archaic forms come to dominate mental life they become the basis of psychopathology.

Psychoanalysis thus seeks to reveal the historical continuities that underlie apparent discontinuities, whether this be at the level of general psychological development or more specifically. For example, those moments of change or transformation that occur in what we term a 'breakdown' often present themselves as impressive discontinuities in mental life. Part of the therapeutic task will be to show that there are continuities occurring, albeit at a less apparent level. This type of understanding not only imparts meaning to symptoms, but goes further as the following illustrates.

Shortly after the death of his father, Mr D developed symptoms that were nearly identical to those his father had suffered. In the course of psychotherapy, it was possible to understand that this expressed his unconscious identification with his father and a way of keeping him alive. However, it was also a way of making himself suffer, thereby expressing the guilt at the painful realisation that he had felt triumph arising from death wishes towards his father.

At one and the same time, this kind of understanding addresses the meaning of the symptom and displays its causal structure and history.[3]

Tom Freeman (1981), a psychoanalyst who worked in a general psychiatric setting, gives the following excellent illustration of an impressive *manifest* break in continuity characterising a psychotic breakdown:

A young man was admitted to hospital in an acute psychotic state. He said to the admitting psychiatrist, 'If you look into my eyes I will betray you'. Freeman learnt from others close to the patient that this overtly psychotic phase had been preceded by an introspective depressive period in which the patient felt worthless and helpless, following a betrayal in love. In this melancholic state, all recriminations against the girl who betrayed him were directed not towards their real target, but towards himself. In other words, the young man, in a typically melancholic manner, identified with his girlfriend (it is he, *not* she, *who is worthless) or, as Freud put it, 'the shadow of the object fell upon the ego'* (Freud, 1917, p. 249). *In this way, he also maintained his idealisation of his lost love. In the next phase, however, a further transformation has occurred: the patient has 'solved' his problem through a psychotic identification. He has* ***become*** *his girlfriend; it is he who is now the betrayer and it is someone else who is the betrayed. The patient resists any restoration of the continuity between the pre-psychotic and the psychotic phase because of the pain it would bring.*

Although there have been very significant theoretical and technical developments in psychoanalysis since Freud's day, the general approach, as outlined here, has not altered.

Personality and illness: a problematic distinction

Psychiatric diagnosis traditionally distinguishes between personality disorder and mental illness. This broad distinction is not without value in terms of forming a general appreciation of the patient and for the purpose of making rational plans for management. Moreover, this differentiation has some importance from an epidemiological perspective, particularly in terms of service planning. For the kind of service necessary for mental illness (which is generally expected to be episodic, although episodes may be very long) is different from that required for the management of personality disorder where there is a reasonable expectation that difficulties will be enduring, even lifelong, given that they are functions of the whole personality structure.

When it comes to the individual, however, the separation between 'personality' and 'illness' is more problematic.[4] In psychoanalysis, illness is always understood in terms of a *personality development* resulting from the stresses of internal and external conditions. Inevitably, individuals have a kind of psychological 'fault line' which, under the pressure of a toxic interaction between a sensitised internal world and particularly malign external circumstances, is brought to the point of breakdown. This fault line, which is often the source of pervasive anxiety, may in other circumstances be managed well enough not to become manifest. A related issue here is that whereas, psychiatrically, one may speak of a patient as having more than one illness, from a psychoanalytic perspective, all the patient's symptoms are seen in a more unitary way, as an expression of his character.

As discussed above (with a different emphasis), a breakdown may *apparently* represent itself as an impressive discontinuity in psychic life but, when examined more carefully, may reveal, in bizarre and distorted form, conflicts and preoccupations that were part of the personality long before the breakdown. In fact, helping the patient integrate his pre- and post-breakdown state is an important part of working analytically with such conditions, as is helping with the less welcome discovery that recovery from the illness is not the same thing as recovery from the difficulties that brought about the illness. These will continue to operate, though at a less manifest level, within the character structure of the individual.[5]

Mr A, an academic, suffered from a severe manic-depressive disorder. When manic, he felt himself to be in possession of a kind of knowledge that was both absolute and his alone; in this state, he believed that he was the object of considerable envy. When depressed, he felt himself to have been ejected from his epistemological paradise and, as an inferior creature, to be the object of everyone's contempt. However, during his so-called 'normal phases', Mr A revealed himself to be still overwhelmingly and continuously preoccupied with his position relative to others (was he bigger or smaller?) or, more precisely, with his relative position or size in the eyes of his primary object. This obsession, which governed all else in his life, was kept hidden in his more normal phases but quickly became evident in his analysis.

Symptoms versus structures

From a psychoanalytic perspective, symptoms are the outward expression of deeper structures. Treatment, therefore, aims at understanding the underlying psychic structures as a more enduring method of alleviating symptoms.

Mr B, a man in his early thirties, presented in an agitated, depressed state. It emerged that he was acutely bereft, having been abandoned by his girlfriend who had chosen his closest friend instead. His disturbance seemed to be a manifestation of an oedipal depression: he felt forced to watch the couple, his friend and his ex-girlfriend, in a state (as he saw it) of continuous pleasure, triumphing over him. Within a few weeks of psychotherapy with a young woman therapist, however, he was 'cured'. He was back at work, functioning well, feeling happy in the world and very far from his depressed state. Indeed, he had a new girlfriend who had herself chosen him over her husband. His sessions were full of long accounts of the virtues of his new girlfriend, related in such a way as to make his therapist feel, as she put it, like an 'irrelevant observer'.

From a symptomatic perspective, the man is cured (an assessment based on a questionnaire or inventory of symptoms would find no evidence of depression), but looking at things more deeply, one can see that the basic structure remains unaltered. The psychic furniture has not changed: there are still three 'chairs', two occupied by a couple and the other occupied by a depressed, excluded party. In his present life, the last chair is now occupied by the husband of his girlfriend, and in his psychotherapy by the therapist, the 'irrelevant observer'. The excluded person is, thus, the target of a projective system which serves to rid the self of unbearable feelings of rejection, now located in a third party. Such a situation is, of course, inherently unstable.

This vignette serves to make a broader point: most patients tend to seek help at a point in their lives when there has been a breach in the ordinary defensive structures which protect them from psychic disturbance.[6] Their most urgent aim is thus to restore their psychic equilibrium in order to be free of unbearable psychic pain. Thus, in the initial phases, the therapeutic situation is often used as an aid to restoration of the original structure, the status quo ante, and this is probably inevitable.[7] Some patients will leave treatment at this point, having accurately perceived that continuing treatment will undermine their defensive structure and threaten them with a return of symptoms. It is only through managing the return of such symptoms within the therapeutic setting, however, that some real and durable protection against further breakdown can be provided.

The role of agency

As described above, from a psychoanalytic perspective, an individual is never only a passive recipient of illness but is always involved in the manifestations of their disorder. This trenches upon the problematic distinction between 'illness' and 'personality', discussed earlier. However, there is here a further issue of some importance. Certain patients, because of the nature of their difficulties, will pressure others into treating them as if they really *are* passive recipients of an illness. This was well illustrated in the first vignette. Mrs A, at least in the early part of the consultation, presented herself as a kind of passive object, but it was not too difficult to break through this self-objectification. There are patients, however, who firmly resist any alternative that tries to engage them in an active way; that is, they welcome self-objectification. Some psychiatric approaches can, unwittingly, collude with this objectification when they seek to treat the illness as if it really could be alienated from the rest of the personality.

Here the language of 'medical treatment' is based on a false analogy with physical medicine. It suggests that an individual's suffering is best considered within the logic of illnesses and their treatment as something done *to* them. It is as if, in just the same way that an antibiotic can attack a streptococcus, an antidepressant can take out a 'depresso-coccus' that has infected the patient or an anti-psychotic can 'target' the psychosis, conveying a kind of biological specificity that, in reality, does not exist. There is no symmetry, as regards nosological categories, between infectious diseases and psychiatric disorders (see e.g., Moncrieff, 2013). I am *not*, however, suggesting that medication is not helpful, only that the symptomatic relief it can provide should not be overvalued in this way, implying as it does that psychiatric disorders have no connection with the personality of the individual.

A multi-level approach

A particular strength of the Fitzjohn's Unit approach is the application of psychoanalytic thinking to the system within which patients find themselves. We attempt to be as sensitive to disturbances at different levels within the system as to disturbance in the patient. Although much of our work is with individual patients, this does not mean that we reductively locate pathology primarily or exclusively in the individual. For psychoanalysis, causality is complex and multi-layered. Every breakdown takes place within the context of human relationships and is always determined by a combination of individual, group, institutional, and wider socio-political structures, though at any given moment, any one of these levels may be more significant than the others.

The psychiatrist Arthur Crisp (1986 personal communication) conducted a simple study illustrating the systemic contribution to psychiatric disturbance on a ward. The ward staff logged, on a daily basis, the number of events of acutely disturbed behaviour. Each incident as it occurred, was, inevitably, attributed to the problems located in the individual patient. However, the log revealed a more systemic causal factor: the number of incidents was found to rise predictably as the day of the ward round loomed, reaching a maximum on that day itself. The general tension and anxiety caused by the approaching round was a major – and until then unrecognised – factor in the disturbances erupting in individual patients.

When our unit receives a referral we need, at times, to consider this broader context. In the same way that a child referred for psychiatric treatment can be understood as being the presenting symptom of a disturbed family, a referred patient may be better understood as the carrier of a disturbance that belongs to an institutional setting, so it might be more appropriate to intervene at that level (perhaps by a visit to the service that has referred the patient). It is not unusual, for instance, for a very helpful and detailed referral letter to end with words such as, 'I am coming to the end of my work in this service' or, 'the unit where this patient has been treated is currently being reorganised' (both indicating more systemic factors that will need consideration).

Mr F was a 38-year old Eastern European man who came from a very severely disturbed background, although he disowned his own knowledge of this. He was admitted to a ward after a series of self-harming incidents, including cutting, overdosing, a serious attempt at drowning himself (requiring resuscitation), and throwing himself in front of a lorry whilst on leave from the ward (resulting in the amputation of his leg). This most recent incident led to his being transferred to a different hospital which was now responsible for his care. The diagnosis was of 'treatment resistant depression'.

Mr F was referred to the Fitzjohn's Unit but, instead of an individual assessment, we decided to consider the broader perspective and offered a consultation to the ward. During the meeting with the ward staff, I learnt that Mr F had been an in-patient for over two years and the staff's capacity to manage him was nearing exhaustion. He was relentlessly negative, saying that he had nothing to live for, that his life was entirely meaningless. Ms L, his special nurse, saw it as her job to persuade him otherwise, but without any success. Special care was provided for the patient on a daily basis.

In discussion, it emerged that there was a 'politically correct' way of talking about him, as someone who was very ill, suffered, was damaged, and needed special care. However, during the consultation it gradually emerged, that there was another much more negative view of him that was difficult to own. As it became possible to talk more freely, staff spoke of the hatred that was stirred up in them. The nurse who was 'specialling' him described how all meetings were arranged by the team, never requested by the patient. The patient would reluctantly agree to come, but would always add, 'If you think there is any point'. The staff felt extremely burdened with the day-to-day responsibility for keeping him alive and found it very difficult when the patient also said he enjoyed being on the ward, that it was 'like being in a hotel'. It also emerged that a number of the nursing staff worried more about this patient than anyone else, and that this worry invaded their personal lives to the degree that even when they were not on duty they thought about him and phoned up the ward to make sure he was still alive. Each of them felt very alone with this worry, as if it was their own very personal responsibility.

The crucial moment came when the senior consultant, Dr J, felt able to describe her distaste at a scene she was frequently exposed to when the patient's wife visited the ward. The couple would caress each other in a sexually exhibitionistic way, in full view of the staff and patients; it was done just sufficiently to make it clear what they were doing, but not so much that it could be censured. We understood this in the following way: the very public, excited 'intercourse' that was displayed by the patient and his wife made manifest the continuous malignant type of intercourse that was taking place between the patient and the staff. That is, Mr F projected his wish to live into the staff, to the degree that they felt continuously responsible for keeping him alive, and, further, this had become a source of addictive excitement for him. The excitement seemed to derive from at least two sources: from being rid of the burden of a wish to stay alive, but also from a perverse triumphant mockery of the staff, in whom that wish was now located.

Mr F belongs to that group of patients who project the wish to live, in this way, into other people. Although some patients feel relieved by this process, which may then allow others to help them, this was not so for Mr F where there was a more malignant relationship. The more the staff owned Mr F's wish to live, the more he was free of it – it was no longer his concern.[8] It is typical of such situations that the staff's capacity to cope is overwhelmed, as anxiety about these kinds of patients invades their personal life. I have known similar situations in which staff members could not even take a holiday for fear that this would result in the patient's suicide.

As we discussed Mr F's situation further, we learnt that the patient's wife had made a formal complaint against the previous hospital: he had been considered well enough by them to be given leave but then made a suicide attempt. We also learnt that six months previously there had been a successful suicide of one of the patients under Dr J's care, resulting in an exhausting inquiry in which some blame was levelled at the ward team, unjustifiably in Dr J's view.

Thus, one can see how different levels within the system – the patient's inner world, his relationships with staff, the recent history of the consultant and her team, the institutional setting, hospital procedures, and broader NHS policy – all interact to produce and maintain this very disturbing situation. In order to provide appropriate care for Mr F, it would be necessary that those looking after him be helped not to have to take full personal responsibility for whether he lives or dies. That is, although they may inevitably end up feeling responsible, it is important that this position not be supported externally.

It is also very important in these situations that no individual member of staff be psychologically isolated with the patient and that the team make sure that they regularly discuss their involvement with him. This can help minimise the splitting processes, for example, where one staff member is idealised and another denigrated, or one staff member is left holding unrealistic hopes for the future of the patient. (For the earliest but still one of the finest discussions of these processes see, Main's (1957) seminal paper 'The Ailment'.)

This more systemic approach was formerly embraced in many quarters by mainstream psychiatry. However, the current context, particularly the marketisation of health which necessarily costs treatments in terms of individual patients, weighs very heavily against consideration of these systemic factors.

Where staff members do become the focus of attention, it is now less often in order to understand or appreciate their role in a system. Instead they become the objects of blame, with accusations frequently being directed at individual members of staff. Without a multi-level understanding, supervision is in danger of degenerating into surveillance, where staff feel less supported and more criticised as untoward incidents are attributed to their individual failings.

It is clear, then, that although the psychoanalytic attitude has not necessarily sat easily with certain forms of psychiatric thinking, it has until recently been able to maintain something of its position in psychiatric institutes and in the teaching of social workers. However, as discussed, things have transformed dramatically in England and Wales over the last decades. The change has not derived from any new discoveries, or even from anything internal to the mental health system, but rather from huge shifts in our cultural and political landscape over the last thirty years. Neoliberalism, which manifests itself as the increasing penetration of the market form into all spheres of life including health care, has led to the near hegemony of a world-view in which society is (mis)understood as an aggregate of individuals, each seeking to satisfy their own needs (Bell, 1997, 2013). This results in the domination of the nomothetic perspective and the consequent industrialisation of human suffering. Inevitably, what is lost is a more complex, ideographic understanding of the individual as a unique being whose suffering occurs within the narrative of his lived life and the human relationships that surround him.

We in the Fitzjohn's Unit, have been swimming against the current, trying to preserve and develop a different way of thinking about mental illness, human subjectivity, and culture in general. One can only hope that with the increasingly critical evaluation of the role of medication in psychiatric disorder, the realisation that the claims for the success of brief therapies have been grossly exaggerated, that there might be a re-recognition that individuals are bio-psychosocial beings embedded in their culture rather than carriers of various diagnostic labels to be placed like objects on 'care pathways' that so alienate them and the staff providing for their care.

Notes

1. This seminar is now led by Francis Grier.
2. Perhaps a word of caution is needed as regards the very term 'biological', as its use here is really a misuse. A biologist is always interested in the interactions between an organism and its natural environment. If she wants to understand what is ailing a tree, she will examine the soil, the climate, the surrounding trees, etc. So, if a 'biological' or 'medical' decision, made in a psychiatric context, is derived solely or entirely from material endogenous factors, then this, in fact, constitutes a parody, or even a perversion, of biology and medicine.
3. I am aware that I am touching on an important epistemological issue that cannot be dealt with here in any detail. For some, meanings and causes are entirely distinct phenomena, whilst for others it is the intertwining of meaning and cause that characterises the human subject. It is this latter view which is consistent with psychoanalysis as discussed here.
4. In the psychiatric literature, there is a growing sense that that the distinction between mental disorder and personality disorder (which underlies the differentiation of axes in DSM-IV) is questionable (for example, Westen et al, 2006).
5. This commitment, to the restoration of continuity to that which appeared to be discontinuous, again manifests the developmental perspective, as discussed above.
6. The popular term for this state is of course a 'breakdown' and in many ways this is quite accurate, as the cause of the disturbance is a breakdown in the capacity to maintain the defensive structure. The consequent state is usually of mixed anxiety and depression and this was the usual diagnosis up to the 1980s, when, instead, many of these cases came to be diagnosed as suffering from depressive disorder. The phenomenology, however, remains the same although the label is different.
7. For an excellent discussion of the subtle but profound effects of this need for psychic equilibrium see, Joseph (1989).
8. Hanna Segal (1993) provides an excellent account of this kind of triumph over the wish to live, making use of clinical and literary material.

Disclosure statement

No potential conflict of interest was reported by the author(s).

References

Bell, D. (1997). Primitive mind of state. *Psychoanalytic Psychotherapy, 10*(1), 45–57. https://doi.org/10.1080/02668739600700061

Bell, D. (2013). *Mental illness and its treatment today.* CHPI. http://chpi.org.uk/wp-content/uploads/2013/12/David-Bell-analysis-Mental-illness-and-its-treatment-today.pdf

Bell, D. & Kleeberg, B. (2013). Very troubled patients. In P. Hobson (Ed.), *Consultations in psychoanalytic psychotherapy.* Karnac.

Freeman, T. (1981). On the psychopathology of persecutory delusions. *British Journal of Psychiatry, 139*(6), 529. https://doi.org/10.1192/bjp.139.6.529

Freud, S. (1905). Three essays on the theory of sexuality. In J. Strachey (Ed.), *The standard edition of the complete works of Sigmund Freud* (Vol. 7, pp. 125–243). Hogarth.

Freud, S. (1907). Obsessive actions and religious practices. In J. Strachey (Ed.), *The standard edition of the complete works of Sigmund Freud* (Vol. 9, pp. 115–127). Hogarth.

Freud, S. (1917). Mourning and melancholia. In J. Strachey (Ed.), *The standard edition of the complete works of Sigmund Freud* (Vol. 14).

Joseph, B. (1989). Psychic change and the psychoanalytic process. In M. Feldman & E. B. Spillius (Eds.), *Psychic equilibrium and psychic change. New library of psycho-analysis* (Vol. 9, pp. 193–202). Tavistock/Routledge.

Lee, S. W., Morley, M., Taylor, R. R., Kielhofner, G., Garnham, M., Heasman, D., & Forsyth, K. (2011). The development of care pathways and packages in mental health based on the model of human occupation screening tool. *The British Journal of Occupational Therapy, 73*(6), 284–294. https://doi.org/10.4276/030802211X13074383957940

Main, T. (1957). The ailment. *British Journal of Medical Psychology, 30*(3), 129–145. [Reprinted in: *The Ailment and other Psychoanalytic Essays*. Free Association Books, 1989.] https://doi.org/10.1111/j.2044-8341.1957.tb01193.x

Moncrieff, J. (2013). *The bitterest pills: The troubling story of antipsychotic drugs.* Palgrave Macmillan.

Segal, H. (1993). On the clinical usefulness of the concept of death instinct. *International Journal of Psycho-Analysis, 74*, 55–61. [Republished in: J. Steiner (Ed.), *Psychoanalysis, literature and war.* Routledge, 1997.]

'When I nod my head, hit it': leadership and followership in the orchestral environment

Lydia Hartland-Rowe

Expanding on an interdisciplinary event that was part of the Tavistock Centenary celebrations, this paper explores experiences of leadership and followership in the orchestral context. Drawing on a sample of literature from a range of sources exploring organisational life in the orchestra including organisational psychology, music education, social semiotics and sociology, and with reference to psychoanalytic and systems psychodynamics frameworks, the paper makes links between experiences of leadership and followership in the orchestra and work in the NHS.

Introduction and background

The Tavistock has a strong tradition of working to participate in and to celebrate areas of activity well outside the mental health or social care sector. Sometimes this has been serious and scholarly; staff publications on the links with art or literature – Hamish Canham on poetry and psychoanalysis (Canham, 2003) or Michael and Margaret Rustin on drama (Rustin & Rustin, 2002), or the design and delivery of a programme of study focussing on the application of psychoanalytic ideas to cultural phenomena. Sometimes it has been more light-hearted, although still drawing on the conceptual frameworks and talents of staff members: from the 3-hour pantomimes of the 1990s featuring the ghost of Bion, for example, (to be found in the open access file 'Five Tavistock Pantomimes'), to the Tavistock farewell songs written and performed for departing colleagues, and even up to the 'zoom' talent show and regular 'zoom choruses' for special occasions during the Centenary year itself. This paper takes as its starting point an event that took place as part of the Tavistock Centenary celebrations and had as its aim the task of exploring experiences of leadership and followership through a dialogue with a specialist practitioner from an unrelated field; the principal percussionist from a major professional opera company.

The event itself was a conversation. Its broad structure, and the thrust of the content, was collaborated and agreed on beforehand; its design was an interview format, aimed primarily at providing space in which experiences and ideas about the reality of leading and following in ordinary daily orchestral organisational life could be shared. The conversation was coloured by anecdote and illustrated with video clips and its purpose was not to analyse but simply to make contact across different professional settings. The aim was not to interpret, but to inform, to connect and hopefully to entertain. The conversation provided insight into key aspects of experience: leadership and followership in the context of the orchestra's musical activity; leadership 'outside the gig'; and the use and abuse of power in orchestral contexts, including the power to hold influence in relation to equalities and diversity.

This paper will explore in more depth some of the themes that emerged from the event, and will draw on interdisciplinary literature from a range of sources, including systems-psychodynamics, in order to make links between orchestral experiences of leadership and followership, and experiences in NHS and other public sector settings.

Building on the centenary event

The themes from the event were broad, and included some discussion about equity of access into the profession, experiences of leading both inside and outside the rehearsal room or concert hall, experiences of leadership in relation to different conductors, and leading and following within ensemble relations. This paper draws on that initial informal, personal and anecdotal conversation in an effort to explore more systematically some of what the very significant literature focussed on the experiences of musicians has to say, and to make links with experiences in NHS contexts.

Stress and working life

Although not an intended theme, what emerged clearly in the discussions leading up to the event, and in some of the examples and anecdotes, was the stress that is present for many musicians, exacerbated of course by the context in which the discussion took place (a year into the pandemic with its consequent impact on the arts community).

A study looking at the experience of psychological stress in British symphony orchestra musicians (Brodsky, 2006), identified six documented sources of stress for orchestral musicians: the work environment (the physical environment); working conditions; social tensions and interpersonal factors; performance anxiety; being subordinate to the will of a (guest) conductor and concerns about the technical challenges of the job. The list is interesting in its own right as a powerful summary of the specific potential burden of stress for musicians, but is also easily translatable into other settings and contexts. It is a reminder that the orchestra is a workplace, and like other workplaces, both is, and is part of, a system that has impact beyond the immediate activity of the group while it is playing music.

Broadly, the aspects of leadership and followership in orchestral life emerging from the event discussion and from the literature reviewed fall into two closely interlinked areas of activity and relationship: those processes taking place when the orchestra is at work playing ('leadership and followership in the musical space'), and those that are part of the wider work system of the orchestra beyond the rehearsal room or concert hall (leadership and power 'outside the gig').

Leadership and power 'outside the gig'

It is hard to know whether to start 'outside' with the wider system, or 'inside' the musical space, and here a systems psychodynamics framework is helpful. As a framework that proposes, to quote Gould, *'that the observable and structural features of an organization – even quite rational and functional ones – continually interact with its members at all levels in a manner that stimulates particular patterns of individual and group dynamic processes*' (Gould, 2006), it tells us that any individual brings into and influences the workplace with their own history, experience, emotionality, expectations and culture – and simultaneously is influenced, consciously and unconsciously by the system in which they are placed, including the wider social and political system. The individual, however unique, is helpfully understood as representative of a system – and the system is representative of what happens within and between individuals, consciously and unconsciously. The orchestra, which relies on individual ability and authority over the instrument, but also cannot function unless it works as a group, is a powerful example of this – but what makes it 'work as a group' has influences from outside the strictly musical space that can go unrecognised. First, then, to explore some of these systemic influences.

Access and education

We started the event conversation with the thorny question of access; who is included, and who excluded from the orchestral music profession. As in the world of psychotherapy, the history in relation to equalities and diversity is perhaps not encouraging. In the UK, access to state provision for music education in the '60s and '70s, and the grant system for higher education, broadened the classical music profession in relation to class – although it seems likely that the cuts to funding for this kind of music education both at school and conservatory level will have an impact on generations approaching or coming into the profession now. In relation to gender, there is some movement from a European picture where many major orchestras had either no women or very few in specific role (i.e. harp players), where in 1970 conductor Zubin Mehta was quoted as saying in a New York Times interview, '*I just don't think women should be in an orchestra. They become men.*' (Klemesrud, 1970, October 18) and where as recently as 2003 a member of the Vienna Philharmonic Orchestra is quoted in 'profil' magazine as saying, '*Three women are already too many. By the time we have twenty percent, the orchestra will be ruined. We have made a big mistake, and will bitterly regret it.*' (Schneeberger, 2003, February 24). An impressive study in 1995 looks at the impact of the changing gender balance across 4 orchestras in Germany, the UK and the USA, with the interesting conclusion that the experience for both the functioning of the orchestra across 5 domains; 'organisational features of the orchestra e.g. 'integrity as an ensemble' and 'player involvement and opportunity'; 'behaviour of the music director e.g. 'direction-setting' and 'coaching'; 'orchestral processes' e.g. 'quality of relationships' and 'musical outcomes'; 'player motivation and satisfaction'; and 'specific satisfactions' e.g. 'job security' and 'compensation'. The research suggested that the experience for women in these contexts was slightly improved when women represented up to 10% of the orchestra, with a steady decline between 10% and 40%, and then, once the balance was closer to 50%, an optimal experience in the domains studied (Almedinger & Hackman, 1995). The authors suggest that it is not clear how much this is unique to the orchestra, how much a pattern in most organisations, and how much part of a wide shift in gender relations. The question framed by the authors is to understand '*what happens when one identity group enters an elite institution that has historically been dominated by another*'; a highly relevant question for our own professions and organisations.

In terms of race and ethnicity, the picture is equally imbalanced, and although there is a rich vein of research into the need to widen access to the classical music profession to be found in American music education journals, there appears to be less to draw on coming from UK sources. One interesting British paper from 2020, focussed specifically on classical orchestral contexts (the primary focus of the Tavistock event and of this paper) acknowledged that players from BAME backgrounds (and women), were able to join the professional music workforce, and were also quite significantly more well-represented in organisations for children and young people (the National Children's and National Youth Orchestra). However, the paper highlights the sustained wider systemic climate of professional performance and broadcast, meaning that the ongoing culture continued to sustain inequity (Griffiths, 2020). Griffiths' research in a sample period showed that 99% of music performed, or broadcast, was by a relatively small pool of male, white composers. The key thrust of the paper was that the adjustments made to some of the practices in the professional orchestra (and educational) environments might have shifted, but that the prevailing exposure through these practices to a long tradition and a network, in company with the weight of the emphasis on a repertoire that had not expanded to be more inclusive, the status quo is maintained. Again, there are resonances with some of the struggles that we face in our professional and organisational contexts, where the way that psychoanalytic psychotherapists are trained, and their own psychoanalysis, is heavily dependent on a lineage of relationships, ideas and practices that can go unacknowledged and therefore unchallenged and unchanged.

Work is clearly going on to make changes; some UK orchestras offer 'Fellowship' schemes aimed specifically at ensuring that players from Black, Asian and minority ethnic backgrounds are encouraged to gain experience and access, and the emergence of the 'Chineke' orchestra in London, which also promotes the wider performance of works by Black composers is a significant development. But it appears that the way in which musicians join an orchestra, whether as a permanent member or as a freelancer, runs all the risks of perpetuating 'the way we do things round here', an organisational climate that is painfully familiar and present for us from 'the snowy white peaks of the NHS' (Kline, 2014). In this country, even if 'blind auditions' are used for orchestral appointments, it is rare for someone to be appointed into an orchestra without a 'trial', where the player rehearses and performs with the orchestra for a period of time as a part of an ongoing process of recruitment. But trials can last months, or even years and still not lead to a permanent appointment. There was in the Tavistock Centenary event discussion a determined emphasis on the idea of the orchestra as a meritocracy, where ultimately the ability to play is all that counts. At the same time, in views also represented in a comprehensive work looking at the meaning of orchestra membership in a 'prestige economy' by Carpos (also a professional musician), there was a recognition that there are other significant factors at work (Carpos, 2017). These factors are often expressed in terms of 'fit', and appear to be more about interpersonal 'fit' than musical capacity, relating more to the many aspects of the orchestral workplace that are about collegiate working. A 2007 paper looking at trust and control in a conductorless orchestra (the New York-based Orpheus Chamber Orchestra describes the system by which players are invited to join the orchestra based on whether or not they are felt to be players who will contribute well to its distributed leadership model – something that is only established by offering them work, or knowing them from working with them elsewhere (Khodyakov, 2007b). The account in the paper suggests that the orchestra members see this as a way of being free of the burden of the organisational power structure of a traditional orchestra, but it is arguable that this way of including new members, with an emphasis on 'fitting in', is not that different. In the event discussion, and in the Carpos paper, musicians speak about the role of and relationship with 'the fixer' (a kind of sub-contractor, also a musician, who works to recruit players on a freelance basis) and what emerges is a clear picture of a system where entry into the organisation depends on a range of capacities and attributes, some transparent and some less so. Success and career progression may depend on this range of influences – perhaps not that far from the recruitment systems being revisited in many NHS organisations, including the Tavistock and Portman, where progression for people from Black, Asian and Minority Ethnic backgrounds, as well as for women (beyond a certain level of seniority) and people with disabilities is not well represented. It is certainly a way of working, in the UK, in the Group Relations field, and one which that community is working to make more transparent, where in both the United States and UK GRC communities efforts are being made to develop processes for recruiting directors and staff more formally, including the development of role descriptions and interview processes At the time of writing, the Tavistock Clinic Group Relations Steering Committee is accepting applications for appointment as Director for one of its three annual GRC's, a first in its history, driven by the desire for greater accessibility and transparency.

There is perhaps another parallel in terms of education, and the place of classical music education in our society and beyond. The music education literature reflects a painful examination of the place of Western classical music, and attitudes to teaching and learning music heavily influenced by that tradition and the cultural, social and political history in which it has evolved and thrived. Two contrasting papers are helpful in highlighting the tensions being grappled with, again with close parallels to the examination within the psychoanalytic community of our relationship to core texts from the past as well as our approach to teaching. In a helpful paper written in the context of the philosophy of music education, Mark Whale explores the complexity of attitudes to Bach in modern music education in relation to a proper consideration of cultural history and context (Whale, 2020). He suggests that to see Bach as only the product of a period in history, with its system of power and oppression, and therefore to relegate or dismiss the study of Bach's music as work which can only be seen in that context and defined by it, is to miss the opportunity and the challenge to relate to Bach's work with rigorous self-reflexivity; that is, to be as interested in *why* we relate in the way we do, coming as we do into listening or playing filled with our own history, culture and pattern of associations. His argument suggests that it is the possible encounter with this challenge that makes Bach as relevant now as ever – the problem is an encounter that is about retreat or comfort rather than ongoing engagement.

This has helpful connections with a way to approach psychoanalytic texts that evolved in a particular cultural context; that is, to be as curious, and rigorous, about our acceptance or our readiness to accept ideas and in the process to use what that history has given us. A complex and challenging paper written in the language of philosophy, Whale's paper works well in parallel with a music education paper (Hess, 2021) that gives more ordinary examples of the ways that music teachers could notice, and challenge racism in the teaching of music, in which vignettes are given of moments in the classroom where either students or the teacher pause to notice the privilege or hidden prejudice in the choice of repertoire, the method of teaching, or the impact of wider events on the experience of students (one example takes place the day after George Floyd's murder). The examples are apparently simple, but are moments of being ready to question accepted knowledge and practice and they are relevant because of the possible parallels with the relationship psychoanalytic psychotherapists have to our history and our practice, and also to highlight the possible differences to the experiences of wider inclusivity that these approaches could make. They also highlight the crucial role of observation or self-reflection in approaching this aspect of experience; being ready to notice the responses of others and our response in return, and being ready to notice what is taking place in our relationship to activity that is meaningful for us, whether it is music or psychoanalytic thinking.

Political and societal contexts

The orchestra exists, like all organisations, in a wider system and a political environment. The impact on music education has already been mentioned; the cost of musical education, and the impact this has on choices for children and young people from lower income backgrounds in the absence of publicly funded music education. The 'El Sistema' project, which originated in Venezuela as a social action initiative aimed at promoting community and leadership capacities in children from severely deprived environments, used group orchestral music-making as a medium for work. It is a project that is the focus for ongoing hot debate, whether in relation to the original and ongoing Venezuelan project or the international initiatives that have followed it, a debate reflected in papers both celebrating it as a model for developing leadership and social action as well as music education, and those offering a robust criticism of the project as a form of colonialism and oppression, and even abuse. Some of the aspirations, and the objections, are about the role of 'El Sistema' in the wider social systems in which it is housed (Baker & Frega, 2018). A study looking in some detail at the work of a Swedish El Sistema-inspired project highlights the small, and significant ways in which the project struggles to find a way to challenge and redress the claims of universal cultural meaning that aspects of the programme could be seen to promote (Bergman et al., 2016). In trying to balance the significant emphasis of the El Sistema model on the value of Western classical music traditions with some recognition of the multicultural profile of the children involved in the project, there is a tension, noted by the authors, that leads inadvertently to enactments of exactly what the project is aiming to avoid. A powerful example is a moment when what the authors describe as a 'dark-skinned child' is singled out from the otherwise largely white orchestra to be interviewed by the compere at a concert – and to stand on her chair to do so. This brought to my mind the tension we face in projects within the psychoanalytic field aimed at encouraging greater access for people from BAME backgrounds; the genuine value, for example, of bursary funding available to students/trainees from these backgrounds and the simultaneous way in which they isolate and separate. The challenge is to work with that tension.

The impact of the wider social and political environment on orchestral life has of course been hugely influenced by the experience of the pandemic, during which the discussion event took place. Even musicians with contracted employment in orchestras were affected, with the freelance community left struggling to manage financially, and divorced from the experience of working and exercising their skill and craft. The vulnerability of the individual musician to the wider economic climate emerges from the literature and certainly in the Tavistock Centenary event the impact of Covid, often career-breaking, was painfully visible. For UK-based freelance musicians, the loss of ease of movement in Europe as the impact of Brexit hits home, is likely to further reduce the opportunities for many individual musicians. But even without the impact of the past 2 years, the literature also points to vulnerability of the orchestra itself, as part of a socio-political environment. Papers exploring the impact of the extended strike of an orchestra in Atlanta (Glynn, 2000) and a study looking at the impact of the experience of musicians in East and West Germany before and after unification, with orchestras from the US and UK featuring as a form of 'control' group also highlight the impact of social and political processes on the experience for professional musicians (Almedinger & Hackman, 1996).

So why go so far away from the relationships at work in the orchestra, as a psychoanalytic psychotherapist writing in a journal for psychoanalytic psychotherapists? Systems psychodynamics thinking, and the practice of group relations, provides powerful evidence for the impact of context on relational intimacy in work contexts, and vice versa. It is clear that the wider systemic factors at work influencing a group of individuals who will join together to rehearse, or to perform, are varied, far-reaching and complex. Experience of and attitudes to leadership and followership are at work in relation to learning, to employment, to working within or shaping and changing orchestral cultures, to managing wider social change. So before the orchestra sits down to play, there will already be, and have been, a network of expectations, ambitions, anxieties connected to practical and emotional aspects of working life that is 'live' and can influence the work of the orchestra in the musical space. It is, of course, tempting and possible to hypothesise on the ways in which such anxiety (unconscious), might hold sway on group functioning in an orchestral setting. Basic-assumption dependency might be at work, for example, when musicians appear not to be listening to each other but relying too heavily on the conductor for the creation of an accurate and clear rendition; or basic-assumption fight-flight might be at work when orchestral management demands from outside the rehearsal room or concert hall are seen as only an intrusion to be avoided or a source of conflict to be challenged (Bion, 1948). It is also possible that the next conductor, the next season, the next soloist might be seen as the solution to the orchestra's problems of survival, in basic-assumption paring mode. But any of these hypotheses would be highly speculative unless based in detailed, careful, respectful observation and testing, and perhaps to be resisted if the orchestra, and the musicians who make up the orchestra, are not to become a proxy client who has neither requested nor authorised treatment or consultancy!

Leadership and followership in the musical space

The work of the orchestra, in the rehearsal or performance space, is a complex collaborative group act, where leadership, followership and both conscious and unconscious motivations and assumptions are at play, as in any group. A move from the wide angle view of the wider system back into the close focus on daily experience may help to bring this to life: an account from the event, of the different ways that a 'rank and file' string player and a principal percussionist might arrive at a rehearsal. The violinist would be booked, would check their diary, make themselves available, make sure they either knew the part or were confident that they would be able to manage it, would make sure they were there in good time, travelling perhaps by bus carrying their fiddle, showing active followership in all of this, and being ready to play and seated in their place with plenty of time. The principal percussionist would get contacted in the same time frame, and would then select and book the rest of the section depending on the repertoire, organise the instruments for which the repertoire is scored, arrange transport for the instruments, ensure the set-up, rush off for a quick cup of tea – and arrive just on time to be met by the violinist's raised eyebrows and a comment that they are 'cutting it fine'. It is an example of the complex leadership and followership roles taken up at times by musicians, beyond the act of playing, and also a familiar example of the risks in any multidisciplinary team where there is a lack of interest or understanding in each others' roles and working realities. If the view of the percussionist as 'not committed' – or a view of the violinist as 'superior and critical' – persists into their working relationship and stops them respecting each others' contribution as players within the musical space, then this will have an impact on the work of the whole group, as with any multidisciplinary team or organisation reliant on different functions and roles. In the act of music-making, the score, the conductor and each musician's authority over their instrument provides clarity about role and task, visible and audible to all if they are watching and listening – but it is much harder to have sight of the whole system at work in all of the other spaces occupied by members of an orchestral community, and it may be in these spaces that tensions arise.

Locations for leadership and followership

The event discussion provided examples of the ways, and places, in which leadership and followership are expressed in orchestral life.

One is the relationship to the beat, lived through the relationship between the conductor and their baton, and the player and their instrument. We were offered different visual and anecdotal examples of the ways that a conductor might 'offer' the beat (i.e. lead) and different ways that the player/s might relate to that offering (i.e. follow). One version of the beat might be so unclear as to throw the musicians onto their own resources, and their capacity to listen to others in order to remain in contact with the score and the task; another might require them to follow with minute attention and go where the baton takes them with precision.

The first example suggests a leader who cannot lead and requires a follower who will work with their lack of capacity, the second a leader who requires a certain kind of followership, a precise and meticulous submission to the leader's vision, authority and practice. The third example is of a kind of mutual leading and following, where conductor and player work together to respond to each other, and where mutual listening and response were central to the work. Examples from jazz ensembles highlighted further the power of the beat, and the choices to be made about how to relate to it; none of them either wrong or right, but different ways of 'following the beat' as determined by the leader of the ensemble or work group.

I wish here to highlight a few papers, from a large and diverse literature, that explore the role of the conductor in the context of leadership, and followership. The first dispenses with the conductor altogether – although not with leadership. It is a study of the Orpheus orchestra based in New York – a conductorless orchestra (Khodyakov, 2007b). The particular focus by the author is on 'trust and control', emphasising the importance for the musicians of feeling able to trust and able to exercise control, and the challenge of working in this way. While there is no doubt that the success of the orchestra does indeed rely on collaborative working, on trust and on shared control, it is also of interest here because of what it suggests about the difficulties that may be associated with the presence of a conductor – what is it that can be eliminated/exported if there is no conductor? It certainly seems probable that aspects of the experience associated with the anxiety deriving from the primary task can be projected into the (absent) conductor, although without this exploration as a specific focus supported by careful 'observation with consent', this can only be speculation. The paper also makes reference to a number of ways in which some delegated leadership and a system for taking authority needed to be developed in order for the orchestra to function and survive as a viable source of income and employment. It also includes some detail about leadership roles that have come into existence and then been eliminated from the structure, some of which involved innovation and income generation. This suggests that the preference may be for limited authority for **any** individual, and shared leadership for all, with leadership and followership roles shifting, albeit according to the authority of a schedule and a structure for representation.

Several studies looking at the role and function of the conductor perhaps suggest the challenges of the followership function in relation to leadership in that role. A picture of the conductor as the source of discipline, inspiration, or an obstacle to or a facilitator of experiences of mutual trust and control emerge from this sample of papers – and these are familiar versions of leadership for anybody who has worked in a managed system, whether leading or following, or, as is more usual, both. For example, a paper written using Foucault as a key influence explores the role of 'discipline' in order to produce art (Sardais et al., 2019) and again, interrogating the role of the conductor and their authority, one of the papers exploring the El Sistema experience looks in detail at a rehearsal process in order to explore the role of the conductor – to empower or to discipline? (Boia & Boal-Palheiros, 2017). A German paper looking at leadership and cooperation has as its core premise the idea that 'charismatic-directive' leadership is what is needed for a conductor to lead a successful orchestra, suggesting a version of leadership and followership that is heavily reliant on the qualities of the leader (Boerner et al., 2004). In a conference paper with a greater focus on collaboration, but still emphasising the qualities needed by the conductor, Khodyakov explores what he calls the 'paradox of the conductor's power' (Khodyakov, 2007a). He identifies a range and balance of qualities that will facilitate collaboration, closing his argument with a paragraph that needs very little translation into other organisational environments:

> (Conductors) should remember that power is a two-way influence process: while conductors decide who is going to be hired and fired, baton-holders have to rely on players' abilities to perform on their instruments and comply with their baton. Such mutual dependency in orchestras is significantly facilitated by trustworthy relationships between conductors and orchestral players. .... They should act as initiators of trust by showing their readiness to empower instrumentalists and allow them to use their talents, skills, and creativity. When musicians view their conductors as being trustworthy, they are more likely to comply with baton-holders' requests and follow their baton even if they do not fully agree with conductors' musical interpretations.

Nearly all of the papers drawn on here include extensive interviews with professional musicians; rich and detailed narratives but coming 'after the fact' of collaborating in rehearsal or performance. They interrogate the relationship between conductor and orchestra from a perspective that firmly identifies leadership and followership as certainly connected to each other, but with a fairly traditional approach to the use of authority and to the nature of the relationship between leader and follower, which may leave something unaccounted for in the complexity of working relationships within orchestral contexts. A paper from an unusual source, social semiotics, provides instead a rich and detailed example of what can inform a powerful and fruitful leadership/followership relationship in the act of playing (Parton, 2014). The methodology is both very different from, but closely connected to a psychoanalytic model of observation, where close attention to detail and sequence allow hypotheses to develop about the nature of the relationships being observed, and the work of development that is unfolding.

Parton describes the work of the orchestra in rehearsal as '*an attempt to align knowledge held by a group of individuals about the interpretation and performance of a piece of music*', and the existence for the orchestra of an 'epistemic domain' holding this knowledge of how the piece should be played. The years of preparation and experience that the members of the orchestra and the conductor bring to the rehearsal means that they can 'gain access', with equal status, to this wider domain of knowledge, but the focus of the rehearsal is to relate to the specific domain '*how this group will play this piece for this performance* '. And here the different relationships and kinds of knowledge come into play, and interact with, and shape each other. Importantly, Parton highlights the significance of the players' knowledge of their bodily experience of playing, and the ways in which this knowledge can be shared and connect with knowledge held by others, including the conductor. She describes the rehearsal, in the context of a relatively rapid pace of work with new repertoire to be rehearsed in a fixed timescale, as the place where musicians share knowledge and find a way to align in relation to the question of 'how to play'. The picture emerges of a working group that has to re-discover in each rehearsal, in relation to the detailed demands for knowledge specific to a particular piece of music (including 'physical' knowledge), configuration of individuals, new relationships to each other's activity, roles and contributions.

There are fascinating parallels with group and organisational functioning here; the need for, and struggle to maintain contact with the 'primary task', and the importance of using knowledge not to obscure or predict (Bion's memory and desire) but to recognise, both in oneself and in others, growing knowledge. But it is in the detailed analysis, written in the language of semiotics and so primarily concerned with the signifiers that communicate knowledge, that a picture emerges of a model for leadership and followership that truly represents the co-creation of new knowledge. There are several examples provided of places where the conductor stops the orchestra playing, and comments on what has happened, and what they have heard. In each of the examples, the language used is a claiming of knowledge, limited only to what he/she can 'know' through what they *hear*, or *can't hear* (rather than what is 'right' or 'wrong'). So all of the work on intonation (whether or not players are all in tune), balance, volume, articulation is initiated by the conductor's sharing of their knowledge of what they can hear, in relation to the knowledge of the musicians. Several exchanges, described in detail from the perspective of the sharing of the 'epistemic stance' taken by all participants, provide a consistent picture of leadership and followership that is working in an interconnected way in order to reach shared knowledge and, literally, optimal performance. The examples include moments where the sharing of his knowledge (something the conductor can hear, or can't hear, or hears a certain way) allows the leader of the orchestra then to share knowledge about the physical reality needed to ensure that 'x' and not 'y' can be heard, and a shared decision is made. As Parton observes,

> the conductor is not using abstract reasonings or invoking scholarly understandings of the work to justify or position his desired changes. Rather, he takes stances on his judgments … which mark such judgments as being based in the moment-by-moment orchestral unfolding exploration of the music work in rehearsal.

She goes on to say,

> [The Conductor] … is demonstrating that he is listening to the Orchestra's playing and is engaging with what they are already producing. He is positioning himself as being 'in the moment' with the Orchestra rather than as a distant, authoritative figure not actively involved in the production of the music performance.

It is this, in Parton's argument, that gives the conductor his authority and allows him to '*achieve change in others' behaviour by achieving change in their state of knowing*'. Although not the focus of the paper, humility and humour, and wider group responses to each other's contributions also emerge from the detailed exchanges, suggesting a level of mutual respect, and the possibility that 'trust and control' are also possible and required within a setting where there is a conductor just as much as where there isn't.

Learning from the orchestra

The model of leadership and followership, and the kind of group interactions that emerge in the example from the Parton paper is one that can lead to new knowledge. It is, in Bion's terms, a Work Group, and no doubt there would be times when even this orchestra, with this conductor, would find itself in more Basic Assumption states of functioning (Bion, 1948). The specificity of the task as defined by Parton '*how will this orchestra play this piece for this performance*?' holds within it so many different variables. If we return to the six stressors in the orchestral workplace identified by the Bronsky study (the work environment; social tensions and interpersonal factors; performance anxiety; being subordinate to a conductor (leader or manager) and concerns about the technical challenges of the job) a whole complex network of possibilities enters the picture. So the balance of individual experience in relation to these stressors, and the nature and weight of unconscious anxiety in the group relating to the challenge of the primary task could, and probably does, at times, shift into a way of functioning that means that the conductor is positioned as someone more authoritarian – or even unnecessary or undesirable.

The example of this orchestra, and this conductor, approaching the task in such a way that each others' knowledge is respected and interacted with, in the interests of together finding the new knowledge needed to do their work, is of course boundaried by a particular task and event. This may seem a long way from the complex organisational work of an NHS organisation. But Parton makes the point early in the paper that '*the professional orchestra ... exists simultaneously as an ensemble of musicians working together to create music, and as an institution concerned with the business of enabling the work of those musicians to occur*'. So the rehearsal will also hold within it the question of the orchestra's survival, its success in the wider context, its future and the future of its members. Perhaps this is no different from a meeting in an organisational context, where different areas of knowledge, practice and experiences need to come together in order to take work forward. How can we develop the capacity in organisational contexts to speak more clearly to the reality of '*what we hear*' – or even to **hear** what we hear when so often the noise coming from inter-professional rivalry and intra-organisational disconnection is so loud? It's entirely possible, even in the Parton example, that there might be a history of this conductor 'knowing' that this second violin section 'always' rushes, or the leader of the orchestra 'knowing' that this conductor 'always interferes' with bowings. Something, in this rehearsal on this day, means that the orchestra and conductor are approaching the task with an open mind, open to each others' knowledge, without these unhelpful versions of each other getting in the way of fruitful collaboration. How often is this something that we manage in an organisational context in a pressed and pressured NHS organisation, where survival is often a constant, and sometimes conscious pressure? Possibly the presence of the researchers, with their openness to fresh knowledge had an influence – which might suggest that the more we can share experience within and across organisations, and be actively exposed to groups and functions that we don't know about, and need to learn about, might be important.

The emphasis on discipline and charisma in some of the other studies suggest a conductor who has to manage or steer a group into a direction that the conductor knows they need to go in, and will either get them there through the strength of their authority or persuade them there through the force of personality. Studies of leadership and followership, as a broad shift, have moved from perspective on leadership that emphasise the qualities of the leader, with their consequent impact on followers, to a perspective on followers in terms of how they relate to certain kinds of leaders – and more recently, to an understanding of leadership as something that emerges from the work that leaders and followers do together.

The Tavistock Centenary event did focus more on some of the difficulties that can be experienced in leadership and followership in orchestral life, with relationships with conductors in particular often featuring miscommunication, misunderstanding or even abuse. We also heard about collaboration and connection between followers, sometimes in spite of a lack of helpful leadership from the conductor and needing to be drawn on in order to protect a performance from disaster, and sometimes engendered and promoted by the conductor finding a way to heighten the players' attentive listening to its highest degree – leading to work of great impact. The fact that the work is making music, which has such emotional impact on human beings, is of course important, but perhaps it has the same status for musicians as the desire to care, or to understand, has for those of us working in what Vega Zagier Roberts defines as 'helping' professions or in psychotherapeutic roles in organisational settings (Roberts, 1994). The workplace is the workplace, and we each bring into it our particular skills and experience, but unless we find ways of relating to each other's contributions with an open mind, ready to 'hear', then as followers, we will struggle to contribute. In the modern NHS organisation in particular, there is a need to listen to a wider range of voices, with equal attention: to voices unrepresented either in our professions or in leadership roles in our organisations, to those providing a range of functions and services, from finance to estates to child psychotherapy; to service users; to students; to the communities in which we are located. It is clearly too big, too complex, and too pressured a system for the ideal model of leadership and followership seen in the Parton example to hold. But there may be some merit in identifying spaces where that way of approaching a shared task could hold, so closely linked as it is to the psychoanalytic stance of 'not knowing'. In 'Memory and Desire' while writing about the challenge to relate fruitfully to what we think we know and what we think we want in analytic work, Bion says that 'it is a matter of trying to get out of the habit of remembering things, and trying to get out of the habit of desiring or wanting anything *while you are predominantly engaged on your work*' (in Mawson, 2018). Perhaps, like the orchestra when it is working collaboratively and with agreed structures for leadership and followership, we can transfer this capacity into our work in the wide organisation and system – where we also, like the orchestra, often face a deadline which is the end of the rehearsal and the need to perform.

Acknowledgments

With thanks to Michael Doran, Principal Percussionist of the English National Opera Orchestra, for joining me in conversation and sharing his experience.

Disclosure statement

No potential conflict of interest was reported by the author(s).

ORCID

Lydia Hartland-Rowe http://orcid.org/0000-0002-7285-2865

References

Almedinger, J., & Hackman, J. R. (1995). The more, the better? A four-nation study of the inclusion of women in symphony orchestras. *Social Forces*, *74*(2), 423–460. https://doi.org/10.2307/2580487

Almedinger, J., & Hackman, J. R. (1996). Organizations in changing environments: The case of East German symphony orchestras. *Administrative Science Quarterly*, *41*(3), 337–369. https://doi.org/10.2307/2393935

Baker, G., & Frega, A. L. (2018). 'Producing musicians like sausages': New perspectives on the history and historiography of Venezuela's El Sistema. *Music Education Research*, *20*(4), 502–516. https://doi.org/10.1080/14613808.2018.1433151

Bergman, Å., Lindgren, M., & Sæther, E. (2016). Struggling for integration: Universalist and separatist discourses within El Sistema Sweden. *Music Education Research*, *18* (4), 364–375. https://doi.org/10.1080/14613808.2016.1240765

Bion, W. R. (1948). Experiences in groups: I. *Human relations*, *1*(3), 314–320. https://doi.org/10.1177/001872674800100303

Boerner, S., Krause, D., & Gebert, D. (2004). Leadership and co-operation in orchestras. *Human Resource Development International*, *7*(4), 465–479. https://doi.org/10.1080/1367886042000246030

Boia, P. S., & Boal-Palheiros, G. (2017). Empowering or boring? Discipline and authority in a Portuguese Sistema-inspired orchestra rehearsal. *Action, Criticism & Theory for Music Education*, *16*(2), 144–172. https://doi.org/10.22176/act16.1.144

Brodsky, W. (2006). In the wings of British orchestras: A multi-episode interview study among symphony players. *Journal of Occupational and Organizational Psychology*, *79*(4), 673–690. https://doi.org/10.1348/096317905X68213

Canham, H., & Satyamurti, C. (Eds.). (2003). *Aquainted with the night: Psychoanalysis and the poetic imagination*. Karnac Books.

Carpos, F. (2017). *The prestige economy of a London orchestra* [Doctoral dissertation]. University College London (University of London). https://discovery.ucl.ac.uk/id/eprint/10024679/1/Carpos_10024737_PhD-E-thesis.pdf

Glynn, M. (2000). When cymbals become symbols: Conflict over organizational identity within a symphony Orchestra. *Organization Science, 11*(3), 285–298. https://doi.org/10.1287/orsc.11.3.285.12496

Gould, L. J. (2006). *The systems psychodynamics of organizations: Integrating the group relations approach, psychoanalytic, and open systems perspectives*. Routledge.

Griffiths, A. (2020). Playing the white man's tune: Inclusion in elite classical music education. *British Journal of Music Education, 37*(1), 55–70. https://doi.org/10.1017/S0265051719000391

Hess, J. (2021). Becoming an anti-racist music educator: Resisting whiteness in music education. *Music Educators Journal, 70*(1), 14–20. https://doi.org/10.1177/00274321211004695

Khodyakov, D. M. (2007a). From a time beater to a music director: The paradox of conductor's power. *Conference Papers – American Sociological Association*. https://eds.s.ebscohost.com/eds/viewarticle/render?data=dGJyMPPp44rp2%2fdV0%2bnjisfk5Ie45PFIr6q1S7Ck63nn5Kx94um%2bSa2ntkewprBKnqq4TbKwsk%2bexss%2b8ujfhvHX4Yzn5eyB4rOvSbOtt0myr7BRpOnnfLum33yxq%2bFJ5KO3ULDaq0zip7dF366xT6vYtk2wr%2bRQ4aiwUK628H3i3%2fE%2b6tfsf7vb7D7i2Lt94uWkjN%2fdu1nMnN%2bGu6myTbersE%2bunOSH8OPfjLvc84Tq6uOQ8gAA&vid=26&sid=0ad35c1f-982d-4d19-a837-b8529f8c2280@redis

Khodyakov, D. M. (2007b). The complexity of trust-control relationships in creative organizations: Insights from a qualitative analysis of a conductorless Orchestra. *Social Forces, 86*(1), 1–22. https://doi.org/10.1353/sof.2007.0100

Klemesrod, J. (1970, October 18). Mehta's mystique: Baton in hand, foot in mouth? *The New York Times*. https://www.nytimes.com/1970/10/18/archives/mehtas-mystique-baton-in-hand-foot-in-mouth-the-hiring.html

Kline, R. (2014). *The snowy white peaks of the NHS: A survey of discrimination in governance and leadership and the potential impact on patient care in London and England* (Project Report). Middlesex University. [Monograph]. https://doi.org/10.22023/mdx.12640421.v1

Mawson, C. (Ed.). (2018). *Three papers of W.R. Bion* (1st ed.). Routledge. https://doi.org/10.4324/9780429454554

Parton, K. (2014). Epistemic stance in orchestral interaction. *Social Semiotics, 24*(4), 402–419. https://doi.org/10.1080/10350330.2014.929389

Roberts, V. Z. (1994). The organization of work: Contributions from open systems theory. In A. Obholzer, & V. Z. Roberts (Eds.), *The unconscious at work: Individual and organizational stress in the human services*. Routledge.

Rustin, M., & Rustin, M. (2002). *Mirror to nature: Drama, psychoanalysis and society*. Karnac Books.

Sardais, C., Lortie, J., & Coblence, E. (2019). Inside the "Panacousticon": How orchestra conductors play with discipline to produce art. *International Journal of Arts Management, 22*(1), 73–85. https://eds.s.ebscohost.com/eds/viewarticle/render?data=dGJyMPPp44rp2%2fdV0%2bnjisfk5Ie45PFIr6q1S7Ck63nn5Kx94um%2bSa2ntkewprBKnqq4TbKwsk%2bexss%2b8ujfhvHX4Yzn5eyB4rOvSbOtt0myr7BRpOnnfLum33yxq%2bFJ5KO3ULDaq0zip7dF366xT6vYtk2wr%2bRQ4aiwUK628H3i3%2fE%2b6tfsf7vb7D7i2Lt94tikjN%2fdu1nMnN%2bGu6exUbGtr1Cyr6R%2b7ejrefKz5I3q4vJ99uoA&vid=31&sid=0ad35c1f-982d-4d19-a837-b8529f8c2280@redis

Schneeberger, P. (2003, February 24). Die Zwei-Prozent-Gesellschaft. *profil Magazine*. English translation available at http://www.osborne-conant.org/profil.htm]

Whale, M. (2020). Talking Bach in an age of social justice. *Philosophy of Music Education Review, 28*(2), 199–219. https://doi.org/10.2979/philmusieducrevi.28

Index

For Product Safety Concerns and Information please contact our EU
representative GPSR@taylorandfrancis.com
Taylor & Francis Verlag GmbH, Kaufingerstraße 24, 80331 München, Germany

www.ingramcontent.com/pod-product-compliance
Ingram Content Group UK Ltd.
Pitfield, Milton Keynes, MK11 3LW, UK
UKHW020203200926
475702UK00004B/588